the Galactagogue Recipe Book

By Frank J. Nice,
RPh, DPA, CPHP
& Myung H. Nice

Lavaun,

Smacznego!
Enjoy (in Polish),
Have fun cooking this healthy stuff.

Frank J Nice

The Galactogogue Recipe Book

Frank J. Nice, RPh, DPA, CPHP
Myung Hee Nice, MS

© Copyright 2014

Hale Publishing, L.P.

1825 E. Plano Pkwy., Ste. 280

Plano, TX 75074

972-578-0400

800-378-1317

www.iBreastfeeding.com

All rights reserved. No part of this publication may be reproduced or transmitted in any form or by any means, electronic or mechanical, including photocopy, recording, stored in a database or any information storage, or put into a computer, without prior written permission from the publisher.

Library of Congress Control Number: 2014905334

ISBN-13: 978-1-9398473-9-3

Disclaimer: Mothers are encouraged to seek treatment from a certified lactation consultant or knowledgeable health professional for low milk supply issues. The information and recipes in this book are intended to supplement the knowledge of mothers and health providers. All recommendations are made without guarantee on the part of the author or Hale Publishing. This information is advisory only and is not intended to replace sound clinical judgement or individualized patient care. The author disclaims all warranties, whether expressed or implied, of this information for any particular purpose.

Dedication

To all mothers who breastfeed their babies and feed themselves. To all fathers who help cook and feed their wives and their children. To all grandparents who cook and feed their children and grandchildren. To our ancestors who cooked ethnic foods they knew were galactogogues that helped support breastfeeding and tasted great, too. Especially to our Polish and Korean ancestors who immigrated to the United States to make our lives better, so we then could make it better for others.

Acknowledgements

I especially acknowledge my parents, Frank, Sr. and Irene Nice, who taught me (Frank, Jr., co-author) how to cook not only great Polish dishes, but also a whole lot of other great tasting recipes. My wife, Myung, learned Polish recipes from me, and now prepares them even better than I do.

I especially acknowledge my parents, Chong Soon and Jung, who taught me (Myung Hee co-author) how to cook great tasting, one-of-a-kind Korean dishes, which my husband, Frank, Jr., can attest.

We acknowledge Lisa Marasco, Lactation Consultant, and Sheila Humphrey, Lactation Consultant, who provided expert and practical advice on choosing herbal and food galactogogues to include in the recipes.

Thank you to all of you in the breastfeeding community who encouraged us to develop this galactogogue recipe book.

Thank you to our children and grandchildren who have breastfed and encouraged us to continue to be active in the breastfeeding community, as we intimately observed and experienced the benefits of breastfeeding.

Foreword

By Sheila Humphrey, BSc, RN, IBCLC
Author of The Nursing Mother's Herbal

The act of cooking is something uniquely human: preparing food with heat and a mixture of ingredients. Wonderwerk cave in South Africa recently revealed the earliest known kitchen. Scraps of charred bones, twigs, and leaves were found in a long ago campfire, evidence of what I hope was a tasty meal.

Our big human brains require a nutrient-dense diet. Cooked food is easier to chew and more completely absorbed. Today, some would argue that raw foods have virtue in our modern world awash with calories. Yet, a nutrient-dense diet is still needed. The human need to eat well is most simply assured by combining a wide variety of minimally processed food ingredients. For babies, human milk provides the most perfect human food and medicine. Then the arguments begin. What is the natural, original, ideal, perfect, best, et cetera diet for the rest of one's life? What do humans really need to eat? So far, what Michael Pollan famously states is what preventative medicine has said for millenia: "Eat Food. Not too much. Mostly plants."

In Ancient Greece, Hippocrates really had it right when he wrote in 2400 BC, "First, do no harm. Second, let food be your pharmacy." He recognized the primary importance of diet to health, perhaps gaining fame where other physicians of his time did not.

Even in antiquity, the earliest physicians recognized the power of diet to improve health. Prescriptions for specific conditions are recorded, many undoubtedly gleaned from old and wise women. To assist women in making more milk, Dioscorides of Ancient Greece suggested chickpeas or barley water with fennel seed. These simple food-based remedies are still considered beneficial. Much later, and after the widespread incursion of tropical spices into the cookery of Europe, Charlemagne wrote in the eighth century that spices are the friend of physicians and the pride of cooks. In his *Handbook of Culinary Spices*, Jim Duke sums it up, 'All spices have folk medicinal reputations, and extracts of most spices have exciting biological activities. All spices have important curative phytochemicals." He would know, having published over 12,000 scholarly articles documenting the use of plants as food and medicines over his long and illustrious career at the USDA. Our ancestors may not have known what was in edible plants that made them useful, or by what mechanism of action they supported life and health, but they wrote down all available knowledge about them as soon as this was technically feasible. This study of edible plants has only accelerated with the development of plant chemistry and nutrition science. Our knowledge of edible plants is our health inheritance. So, dear readers, please allow for a short trip through the history of plant chemistry. And it is a very short history.

It was just over 200 odd years ago that plant chemists started taking apart plants to discover what chemicals were in them. In 1803, morphine was the first chemical isolated from a plant. It was later discovered to be the 'active ingredient' in opium poppy that relieved pain. Yet it was only in the 1970s that the discovery of opiate receptors in our brains provided a location where morphine acts with it's well-established pain-killing result.

Likewise, consider Vitamin C. In times of food scarcity, scurvy grass was known and used by country folk in England to prevent or treat scurvy. Medical doctors of the time were loath to suggest anything so simple, inexpensive, and local as a common seaside weed, and their patients paid and suffered for it. It took medical researchers a very long time to find what was in fresh foods that made the difference. Even after the British Navy had the proof that limes could prevent scurvy (in the 18th century), sailors still sometimes suffered this disease almost into the 20th century. Then in 1930s came the isolation and testing of the very simple chemical in fresh food, ascorbic acid or Vitamin C, a magic bullet that was found to prevent or cure scurvy. The scientists also found a substance in Vitamin C-rich citrus fruits that they called Vitamin P. Plant chemists had a harder time with Vitamin P, and it was soon found to be a confusing complex of many plant chemicals and researcher interest flagged. No magic bullet there.

The discovery of the B vitamins, such as thiamine and niacin, in commonly consumed whole grains opened the door to modern food science. Processed food staples, such as white flour and rice, were found utterly deficient in these vitamins, the price paid for making these foods stable. Refining grains rendered them inert and non-nutritious to humans, other than as calories. Nothing else would grow on them. Unfortunately, a short-term solution was used that avoided having to re-educate the population on the need to eat whole grains. Today, for example, beriberi and pellagra are very rare in the USA because white flour and white rice are 'enriched' with thiamine and niacin. But with better food labels, we can read for ourselves how whole grains and other cereal seeds are much superior sources of not just B vitamins, but fiber, minerals, and choline as well. And these are just the known 'essential nutrients.' What else could be missing that we have yet to discover?

Plant chemistry exploded as a science in the 1960s, as researchers around the world developed the tools and methods needed to peek inside our heritage of foods and medicinal plants. Plant chemists have now isolated hundreds of thousands of different constituents that naturally occur in plants and have made a start on studying their biological effects. And finally, nutrition science has become inspired to look beyond protein, fats, vitamins, minerals, and fiber to explain why a diet of fruits, vegetable, whole grains, and legumes does a body more good than vitamin pills. The fortunes of the misunderstood Vitamin P have risen; this complex of plants constituents found in Vitamin C-rich foods is now understood to amplify and extend the health actions of Vitamin C, positively influencing a whole host of metabolic processes going on in our cells. The whole orange is SO much better for you than even a mega dose Vitamin C tablet. Of course, as each new plant constituent is discovered to have miraculous properties, the dietary supplement industry and food engineers seize upon this information as manna in the desert. A new marketing opportunity is created: processed food packages start featuring this latest wonder nutrient, and a host of dietary supplements containing the new miracle flood the internet.

Yet, the more researchers examine foods eaten in or near to their original packaging in plants and animals, the more profound benefits they find to protect against our illnesses of modern life. No magic bullets here. The research finds the most benefits come to those who eat a variety of good, wholesome food, mostly plants, and the more varied the better. For clarity, a varied diet means eating a lot of different plants (and animals), not a lot of different ways to eat the same plant. For example, an unvaried diet of wheat products, such as bread, bagels, cookies, pizza, and biscuits eaten day in and day out, leaves no room for all the good things found in other grains and seeds: barley, rice, rye, quinoa, or teff. Variety means eating broadly across the edible plant (and animal) world. Fifty years ago, the founding mothers of La Leche League stated that a variety of foods eaten close to their natural state helped breastfeeding mothers. Food really can be your medicine.

Prevention and the healing of illness require eating a variety of nutrient-dense foods. Yet modern pharmaceuticals can be important for health, too, and should be taken when needed, preferably in consultation with a doctor who is knowledgeable about modern nutritional science. Neither medications nor medicinal herbs work well without a good diet to support their actions. So beware of the wish that a single food constituent, taken by itself in a pill, will fix a health problem all by itself. There is no point in taking lycopene pills to prevent cancer if your plate is filled with charbroiled steak. Where are your vegetables going to fit? Now, just for clarity, I love steak, just not very often, and most of my plate is first filled with salad.

Eating processed foods with expensive supplements is much more expensive than just learning how to cook real food from scratch. While all foods in an ultimate sense support life, some are better at it than others. To help the shopper, I would suggest that real food, that is, food containing most of its original nutritional content intact, be labeled 'natural.' Real food is recognizable as food: fruits, vegetables, herbs, spices, grains, nuts, legumes, meats, fish, and eggs. Food products that have been treated and massaged beyond recognition, losing most of their essential nutrient constituents along the way to the grocery shelf, deserve to be labeled as 'processed,' the easier for the consumer to limit in their diet. Once home from the store with real food, many consumers used to eating a lot of processed foods will need to learn how to cook real food from scratch. So, a recipe comes in very handy indeed.

Recipes are wonderful inventions. You can inherit them, discover them in old cookbooks, keep them a family secret, collect them, publish them in your own cookbook, and now instantaneously steal or share them with the world online. In the history of the recipe, particularly tasty or healthful combinations of foods or herbs were treasured and passed down, and written down for posterity as soon as writing was invented. Three thousand years ago in Ancient Mesopotamia, the earliest written recipe was carefully inscribed on the walls of the tomb of Queen Puabi of Ur. This recipe for flatbread may have recorded a secret and sacred method of preparing mixed grains for later beer brewing. The recipe includes the addition of aromatic herbs for flavor, and perhaps preservation and added health benefit.

Within a few hundred years, the Sumerians were recording recipes on clay tablets, with recognizable plant-based food you may have in your kitchen: onions, garlic, barley, ancient wheat, chickpeas, beans, and a dizzying number of fruits we still love to eat. Interestingly, many of the food plants first cultivated in the Tigris and Euphrates valley are regarded as galactogogues, helpful in making more milk.

A recipe is a little gift through time that recalls a particularly effective herbal remedy or a particularly tasty meal or beverage. Of course, opinions vary on what works or tastes good! With the advent of the printing press, books started to be published that provided instruction to the housewife on the preparation of not only meals, but of herbal remedies. Even today, the word recipe is used for both. Home was also the hospital, so herbal remedies and convalescent recipes (featuring marshmallow, whole grain gruels, and eggs) were standard sections and much relied on. Home remedies and home cooking are still very much a tradition, even in this modern world. Making food and remedies from scratch allows you a profound connection to what you are eating as it educates the palate.

Food is generally something we find tasty and pretty easy to eat. Medicine, not so much, and this is probably for the good. Many medicinal herbs are also foods and taste good, but some are purely medicinal in use and often do not taste good. Pay particular attention to taste when you are pregnant. Be informed about the medicinal dose and appropriate use of any herb that is not used as food. Interestingly, many foods and herbs that are thought to interfere with pregnancy also taste repellent when pregnant. Encountering the real food allows you the chance to smell or taste it more completely, a safety taste test if you like. A Lebanese friend of mine shared a recipe for a dip using soaked fenugreek seeds, ground up with garlic, onion, cilantro, and ginger. She found that while pregnant she could not eat this most beloved of snacks. Coffee lover that I am, its lovely smell was repellent to me as soon as I was pregnant. Espresso regained its divine aroma the day after my daughter was born.

In general, the more medicinal, strong-acting plants taste bitter or acrid, so herbal recipes often include very tasty ingredients to 'help the medicine go down.' Sometimes the taste makes the remedy work, bitters before meals, for example, stimulate gastric juices and improve digestion.

At the other end of the spectrum are the sweets - what humans love to eat. For millennia, we had to eat sweets sparingly; honey, maple syrup, and dates were luxury treats for special occasions. Our all too familiar candy, cakes, and cookies are mostly modern recipe innovations inspired by the extraction of white sugar from sugarcane and sugar beets. In between pure medicine and pure treat is the wonderful idea that sometimes we can have our cake and eat it too: the so-called functional foods. These can be described as foods that are excellent or good sources of essential nutrients (excellent being 20% or more of the daily requirement for an essential nutrient, such as a vitamin, iron, folate, calcium, potassium, magnesium, or choline or fiber; good being 10%). These foods mercifully add zest to our meals: aroma, texture, flavor, and color. I call these the foods the rest of the world eats. Old and ethnic recipe books are filled with scratch recipes using such nutrient-dense, plant-based ingredients, including the aromatic and medicinal herbs and spices, brightly colored fruits and vegetables, all packed with vitamins and minerals, as well as a fabulous array of plant constituents that do a body good.

In the history of cookbooks, I do not believe there has ever before been a book of recipes for the breastfeeding mother, featuring herbs, spices, and foods traditionally used to support milk supply. Frank Nice's book shows how even ordinary-appearing recipes use galactogogues, or foods considered helpful in increasing milk. He has collected recipes from around the world that feature galactogogue spices, such as fennel, cumin, coriander, and fenugreek, and liberal amounts of garlic, in combinations that are tasty and powerfully anti-inflammatory. We could all do with these foods in our daily diet. His Polish recipe for borscht is an interesting example: his family recipe is a nutrient-dense soup that will really help mothers get their choline requirement for the day (nursing mothers need 550 mg choline per day which a typical American diet does not provide). The best part: we certainly don't need to know all the individual 'active' ingredients or what mechanisms of action these food constituents may employ for the nursing mother to get benefit from these foods. In good food, the nutrients work together for amplified healthful effects. Paraphrasing the approach of Chinese Traditional Medicine - that which is good for the mother is good for her milk supply. Frank Nice's cookbook is not a prescriptive approach. It is more an everyday way to improve and diversify the diet. That alone will help make milk. For nursing mothers leading modern stress-filled lives, this collection of recipes offer real nutritional support; the recipes use mostly inexpensive food easily found in most grocery stores, and are simple to prepare. A variety of food. Colorful food. Made with real ingredients: no prepackaged ingredients, no artificial anything. And most importantly, tasty food. This recipe collection invites the exploration of new tastes from around the world, a deepened appreciation for our ancestor mothers who saved the recipe, and an opportunity to have fun in the kitchen.

Table of Contents

Introduction 25
- Major Galactogogues 26
- Minor Galactogogues 27
- Summary 30

Recipes 33
Alfalfa 35
- **Appetizers** 36
  - Deviled Eggs 36
- **Breads** 36
  - Vegetable Pizza Bread 36
- **Salads** 37
  - Asian Noodle Salad 37
  - Avocado Shrimp 38
  - Tossed Salad 39
  - Herb Dressing 39
- **Soups** 40
  - Red Borscht Soup 40
- **Entrees** 40
  - California Chicken Roll 40
  - Chicken Tacos 41
  - Korean Cold Spicy Noodles (Bibum Myun) 42
  - Roast Beef Sandwich 42
  - Shrimp Sandwich 43
  - Smoked Turkey Asparagus Melt 44
  - Tuna Burgers 44
  - Veggie Burgers 45

Anise 47
- **Salads** 48
  - Crab Salad 48
- **Entrees** 49
  - Anise Turkey Curry 49
  - BBQ Sichuan Pork Ribs 50
  - Braised Beef Short Ribs with Anise and Ginger 51
  - Cheesy Anise Chicken 52
  - Chinese Braised Oxtails with Root Vegetables 52

- Oriental Chicken ... 53
- Smoked Pork Loin ... 54
- Tuna Noodle Casserole ... 55

Sides ... 55
- Zucchini with Anise ... 55

Desserts ... 56
- Anise Cookies ... 56
- Blueberry Biscotti ... 57
- Orange Anise Cake ... 58
- Pizzelles ... 59

Beer (Barley/Hops) ... 61

Appetizers ... 62
- Beer Battered Onion Rings ... 62
- Beer Battered Pickles ... 62
- Ranch Dipping Sauce ... 63
- Beer Cheese Spread ... 63

Breads ... 64
- Apple Cheddar Beer Bread ... 64
- Beer Bread ... 65
- Condiments ... 65
- Beer Bacon Spread ... 65

Soups ... 66
- Beer Cheese Soup ... 66

Entrees ... 67
- Beef Beer Chili ... 67
- Beer Battered Prawns ... 68
- Beer Brats ... 69
- Beer Grilled Pork Chops ... 70
- Beer Marinated Pork Chops ... 70
- Braised Beef Shank and Vegetables in Beer ... 71
- Italian Style Beer Battered Seafood ... 72

Sides ... 72
- Spicy Rice with Beer ... 72

Caraway ... 75

Breads ... 76
- Caraway Cheese Muffins ... 76
- Sourdough Rye Bread (Rolls) with Caraway Seeds ... 77

Sourdough Bread 77
Salads **78**
  Caraway Coleslaw 78
  Sauerkraut Salad 79
Soups **79**
  Roux Soup 79
Entrees **80**
  Beef Cabbage Rolls 80
  Beer Beef Stew 82
  Eggplant and Chickpea Stew 83
  Pork Shoulder with Sauerkraut and Apples 83
  Sausage and Apple Rolls 85
  Garlic Butter 86
Sides **86**
  Cheesy Fried Rice 86
  Ginger Garlic Paste 87
  Garam Masala (or store bought) 87
  German Style Red Cabbage 88
Desserts **89**
  Caraway Cake 89

Chasteberry 91
Beverages **92**
  Chasteberry Tea 92
Salads **92**
  Fruit Salad with Chasteberry Dressing 92

Coriander 95
Appetizers **96**
  Deviled Egg Dip 96
Salads **96**
  Avocado Grapefruit Salad with Coriander Dressing 96
  Cabbage Salad 97
Soups **98**
  Brown Lentil Soup 98
  Carrot Sweet Potato Soup 99
Entrees **100**
  BBQ Pork Spareribs 100
  Coriander Lemon Chicken 101
  Creole Chicken Livers 101

Fish Tacos with Lime-Cilantro Salsa 102
Marinated Prime Rib Roast 103
Moroccan Stuffed Potatoes 104
Baharat Spice Mix (or you can use store bought) 106
Slow Roast Pork 106

Sides 107
Spiced Butternut Squash 107

Dandelion 109
Condiments 110
Dandelion Honey 110

Salads 110
Blue Cheese Dandelion Salad with Citrus Dressing 110
Dandelion Greens with Pennsylvania Dutch Hot Bacon Dressing 111

Soups 112
Hearty Vegetable Soup 112
Spring Vegetable Soup 112

Entrees 113
Creamy Dandelion Greens and Ham 113
Linguine with Dandelion Greens 114
Marinated Chicken with Spinach and Dandelion Greens 115
Pasta with Dandelion Greens and Ricotta 116
Pasta with Dandelion Stems 116
Ravioli with Dandelion and Fenugreek 117

Sides 118
Batter Fried Dandelion 118
Creamed Dandelion Leaves 118
Dandy Dandelions 119
Pennsylvania Dutch Dandelion Greens 120

Dill 121
Breads 122
Dill and Scallion Batter Bread 122
Yogurt Dill Biscuits 123

Condiments 123
Dill and Yogurt Salad Dressing 123
Polish Dill Pickles 124

Salads 124
Arugula with Pears and Dill 124
Cucumber Dill Salad 125

  Dill and Cucumbers in Sour Cream Dressing 125
  Dill and Shallot Potato Salad 126
  Shrimp and Shell Pasta Salad 126
  Zucchini Dill Salad 127
 Soups **128**
  Sweet and Sour Cabbage Soup 128
 Entrees **129**
  Beef Gyros with Dill Sauce 129
  Beef Sirloin/Tenderloin Stroganoff with Dill 130
  Meatballs with Dill Dressing 131
  Reuben Sandwich 132
  Salmon with Mustard Dill Sauce 132
 Sides **133**
  Creamed Pumpkin with Dill 133
  Potatoes Gratin with Dill 134

Fennel **135**
 Appetizers **136**
  Fennel Fritters 136
  Meatballs with Fennel Sauce 136
  Fennel Sauce 137
 Bread **138**
  Fennel Blue Cheese Flatbread 138
  Greek Seasoning 139
  Fennel Tea Biscuits 139
 Salads **140**
  Beet Fennel Salad 140
  Fennel Cumin Flank Steak Salad 140
  Mushroom Fennel Salad 141
 Soups **142**
  Potato Fennel Soup 142
 Entrees **143**
  Chicken Pot Pie with Mushrooms and Fennel 143
  Fennel Stuffed Sea Bass with Broccoli 145
  Mussels in Fennel Sauce 146
  Oriental Chicken Stir Fry 146
  Seared Chicken with Mashed Fennel 147
  Crispy Leeks 148

  Slow Roasted Pork with Fennel, Tomatoes, and Olives................................148
 Sides 149
  Roasted Butternut Squash and Fennel...149

Fenugreek 151
 Beverages 152
  Fenugreek Tea 152
 Breads 152
  Fenugreek Flatbread..152
  Condiments..153
  Jamaican Curry Powder..153
  Tomato Chutney 154
 Soups.. 155
  Butternut Squash Soup 155
 Entrees 156
  Asian Crusted Salmon...156
  Fenugreek Cashew Chicken 157
  Onion Paste 158
  Garlic Paste 158
  Cashew Nut Butter..158
  Fried Chicken Liver 159
  Leftover Turkey/Chicken Curry...160
  Oven Baked Herring 161
 Sides 161
  Deep Purple Potatoes 161
 Desserts 162
  Saint Hildegard Cookies 162

Garlic... 165
 Appetizers 166
  Garlic Hummus..166
  Tahini..166
 Soups.. 167
  Black Bean Soup 167
  Garlic and Poached Egg Soup 168
  Nice Polish White Borscht 169
  String Bean Garlic Soup..170
 Entrees 171
  Baked Spaghetti Casserole..171
  BBQ Boneless Chicken Breast..171

  Beef Stew 172

  Garlic Balsamic Halibut or Sea Bass 173

  Glazed Pork Chops 173

  Lasagna 174

  Prime Rib with Horseradish Sauce 175

  Horseradish Sauce 176

  Yankee Chili 176

  Zucchini Soufflé with Garlic Croutons 177

  Garlic Croutons 177

 Sides **178**

  Garlic and Herb Mashed Potatoes 178

  Garlic Quinoa 178

  Sautéed Brussels Sprouts 179

Goat's Rue 181

 Beverages **182**

  Goat's Rue Tea 182

Marshmallow Root 183

 Desserts **184**

  Chocolate Mousse with Marshmallow Root Fluff 184

  Marshmallow Root Marshmallows 184

  Rose Water 185

  Marshmallow Root Meringue 186

  Chocolate Sauce (double recipe, if also dipping) 186

  Original Marshmallows 187

  Toasted Coconut Marshmallow Ice Cream 187

Oats, Oat Straw, Oatmeal 189

 Beverages **190**

  Oat and Mango Smoothie 190

 Breads **190**

  Cherry Blueberry Oat Muffins 190

  Pineapple Raisin Oat Bran Muffin 191

  Strawberry Jam Oat Squares 192

 Breakfasts **192**

  Oats Cereal 192

  Oatmeal Pancakes 193

  Oatmeal with Vanilla Soy Milk and Fresh Berries 193

 Soups **194**

  Oatmeal Chicken Soup 194
 Entrees **195**
  Oat Battered Fried Chicken with Garlic Mayonnaise 195
  Oat Crusted Chicken with Dill 196
  Turkey Meatloaf 196
  Zucchini Quiche 197
 Desserts **198**
  Apple Custard Pie 198
  Black Cherry Crumble 199
  Chocolate Banana Oat Cake 200
  Chocolate Banana Peanut Butter Oatmeal Cookies 201
  Crockpot Apple Crisp 202

Quinoa 203
 Salads **204**
  Hijiki Salad 204
  Quinoa and Dill Salad 205
  Quinoa, Chickpea, and Kale Salad 206
  Sweet Potato Quinoa Cakes on Salad Greens 207
  Avocado Dressing 208
 Soups **208**
  Quinoa Hearty Galactogogue Vegetable Soup 208
 Entrees **210**
  Baked Quinoa Casserole with Potatoes and Cheese 210
  Quinoa, Lima Bean, and Corn Casserole 211
  Quinoa Patties with Mustard Dill Sauce 212
 Sides **213**
  Quinoa with Carrots, and Peas 213

Red Clover 215
 Beverages **216**
  Herb Tea 216
  Red Clover Lemonade 216
  Red Clover Tea 216
 Breads **217**
  Red Clover Corn Bread 217
 Condiments **218**
  Red Clover Jelly 1 218
  Red Clover Jelly 2 218
 Salads **219**

  Red Clover Spinach Salad 219
 Entrees 220
  Asian Noodles 220
  Red Clover Burritos 221

Red Raspberry 223
 Beverages 224
  Red Raspberry Tea 224
 Condiments 224
  Red Raspberry Honey Vinegar 224
  Red Raspberry Jam 225
  Red Raspberry Vinaigrette Dressing 225
 Salads 226
  Salad with Red Raspberry Vinaigrette Dressing 226
 Entrees 226
  Grilled Lamb with Red Raspberry Sauce 226
  Basil Pesto 227
  Red Raspberry Sauce 227
  Red Raspberry Glaze No. 1 228
  Red Raspberry Chicken 229
  Red Raspberry Glaze No. 2 229
 Desserts 230
  Peach Dumplings with Red Raspberry Sauce 230
  Red Raspberry Cobbler 231
  Red Raspberry Cheesecake 231
  Red Raspberry Oatmeal Bars 232

Stinging Nettle 233
 Beverages 234
  Stinging Nettle Tea 234
 Soups 234
  Dandelion Nettle Soup 234
  Irish Stinging Nettle Soup 235
  Stinging Nettle Soup 1 235
  Stinging Nettle Soup 2 236
 Entrees 237
  Gnocchi Verde (Green Dumplings) 237
  Ravioli with Stinging Nettle Sauce 238
  Stinging Nettle Sauce 238
  Stinging Nettle Mashed Potatoes 239

Stinging Nettle Pasta 240
　Sides **240**
　　Stinging Nettle Custard 240
　　Stinging Nettle with Nuts 241

Thistles 243
　Beverages **244**
　　Blessed Thistle Tea 244
　　Milk Thistle and Red Raspberry Smoothie 244
　　Milk Thistle Seed Tea 245
　Breakfasts **245**
　　Milk Thistle Muesli 245
　　Milk Thistle Porridge 246
　Condiments **246**
　　Milk Thistle Condiment 246

Vervain 249
　Beverages **250**
　　Vervain Mint Tea 250
　　Vervain Tea 250
　Desserts **250**
　　Peach Vervain Tart 250

References 253
Index 255
About the Authors 257
Ordering Information 259

Introduction

A good human milk supply for newborns and infants in past times was crucial for survival. Historically, it is evident that nations, cultures, and tribes developed traditions based upon herbs and foods being used to maintain and increase milk supply. Today, mothers continue to be concerned about inadequate quantity of breastmilk. Many patients will attempt to increase the quantity of their breastmilk production by taking herbs and foods called "galactogogues." These substances increase milk supply, likely by increasing prolactin or oxytocin to initiate the breastmilk letdown reflex and aid in breastmilk ejection.

Common herbs and foods used as galactogogues are numerous and various, and have included: alfalfa, almonds, anise, asparagus, barley, basil, beets, caraway, carrots, chaste tree fruit, cherries, chicken broth/soup/stock, chickpeas (garbanzo beans), coconut, coriander seeds, cumin, dandelion, dill, fennel, fenugreek, flax seeds, garlic, ginger, goat's rue, green beans, hibiscus, hops, lemon balm, lentils, lettuce, marshmallow root, millet, molasses (black strap), mung, mushrooms, nettle, oat straw (oats), papaya, peas, pumpkin, quinoa seeds, red clover, red raspberry, rice, sage, seaweed soup, sesame seeds, spinach, sunflower seeds, sweet potatoes, thistles, turmeric, and vervain. Many continue to be used by breastfeeding mothers and are recommended by mothers, grandmothers, lactation consultants, and healthcare professionals (Humphrey, 2003; Humphrey, 2007; Marasco, 2008; Nice, Coghlan, and Birmingham, 2000).

As with prescription drugs and over-the-counter (OTC) medications, breastfeeding women use herbals to treat a variety of ailments and to maintain health. Herbal use is as prevalent among breastfeeding women as it is with consumers who are not breastfeeding. Herbals provide the opportunity not to use a prescription or OTC medication. In fact, lactation consultants recommend and breastfeeding mothers take galactogogues to help increase milk supply. Major galactogogues (galactogogues that are most commonly used as a single therapy) include: chaste tree fruit, fennel, fenugreek, garlic, goat's rue, and thistles. Minor galactogogues (galactogogues that are not used as often as major galactogogues and tend to be used more often in combination therapy) include: alfalfa, anise, borage, caraway, coriander, dandelion, dill, hops, marshmallow root, nettle, oat straw, quinoa, red clover, red raspberry, and vervain. Miscellaneous galactogogues include all others not classified as major or minor.

Most knowledge about herbal use during breastfeeding and potential side effects of the wide variety of herbals used as galactogogues comes from the systematic collection of data in Germany — the *German Commission E Monographs*, which have been translated into English (Blumenthal, Busse, Goldberg, & Gruenwald, 1998). There are also several published texts that provide useful information on herbal use during breastfeeding. These include *The Nursing Mother's Herbal* (Humphrey, 2003), *Nonprescription Drugs for the Breastfeeding Mother* (Nice, 2011), *Medications and Mother's Milk* (Hale, 2012), and PDR *for Nonprescription Drugs, Dietary Supplements, and Herbs* (2011).

Information provided on the use of galactogogues presented in this book can serve as general guidelines for nursing mothers. Major and minor herbal and food galactogogues are covered (Humphrey, 2003; Nice et al., 2000; Blumenthal et al., 1998; Nice, 2011; Hale, 2012; PDR, 2011). This list is not inclusive, but does include the most commonly used nonprescription medicinal galactogogues in the United States. Generally accepted doses of the herbal plants as used in herbal medicine are provided in the list. Note that several different parts of the same plant can be effective as galactogogues. The culinary amounts of herbs in the recipes correspond to the medicinal doses of the herbs.

Major Galactogogues

Blessed Thistle (Cnici benedicti herba)
Medicinal Dose: Up to 2 grams in capsule form daily

Other Uses: May increase appetite and settle upset stomach

Caution: Blessed thistle may cause allergic reaction.

Chaste Tree Fruit, Chasteberry, Vitex (Agni casti fructus)
Medicinal Dose: 30 mg to 40 mg daily as an alcoholic extract (50%-70% alcohol)

Other Uses: To treat breast pain dysmenorrhea

Caution: Herb may cause rash; extract form has high alcohol content, although amount consumed is very small.

Fennel (Foeniculi fructus)
Medicinal Dose: 5 grams to 7 grams daily

Other Uses: For gastrointestinal disorders and as an expectorant

Caution: Fennel may cause allergic reaction and dermatitis.

Fenugreek (Foenugraeci semen)
Medicinal Dose: Orally, 6 grams in capsule form daily

Other Uses: To stimulate appetite, externally to control inflammation

Caution: Fenugreek may cause nausea and vomiting in mother and diarrhea in baby; may increase asthma symptoms or lower glucose levels in mother; may cause skin reactions with external use (avoid nipple area); may cause "maple syrup" smell in mother's and/or baby's urine and/or sweat; do not use if allergic to peanuts and/or legumes.

Garlic (Allii sativi bulbus)

Medicinal Dose: 4 grams to 9 grams in capsule form daily

Other Uses: For possible positive cardiovascular effects and/or immune system stimulation

Caution: Garlic may decrease nursing time due to odor in breast milk, which some babies may not like.

Goat's Rue (Galegae officinalis herba)

Medicinal Dose: 1 mL to 2 mL of tincture, two to three times a day; 425 mg capsules three to four times a day

Other Uses: To lower blood glucose levels

Caution: None.

Milk Thistle (Cardui mariae herba)

Medicinal Dose: 12 grams to 15 grams daily as infusion (equal to 200 mg to 400 mg of silibinin)

Other Uses: For possible liver protective properties

Caution: Milk thistle may have laxative effect and/or cause allergic reaction.

Minor Galactogogues

Alfalfa (Medicago sativa)

Medicinal Dose: Up to 60 grams daily (one to two capsules four times a day)

Other Uses: Diuretic and laxative

Caution: Alfalfa may cause loose stools and/or photosensitivity; do not use if allergic to peanuts and/or legumes; do not use in patients with systemic lupus erythematosus (SLE).

Anise (Anisi fructus)

Medicinal Dose: 3.5 grams to 7 grams as tincture or tea, five to six times a day

Other Uses: For anxiety and as antiflatulent

Caution: Anise may cause allergic reaction.

Barley (Hordeum vulgare)

Medicinal Dose: 15 grams of barley extract; one to two cups of tea daily; one bottle of beer daily

Other Uses: For nutrition and aid to digestion

Caution: None.

Caraway (Carvi fructus)

Medicinal Dose: 1.5 to 6 grams daily as tincture, tea, or essential oil

Other Uses: For anxiety and as antiflatulent

Caution: Avoid large amounts of the essential oil form.

Coriander, Cilantro (Coriandri fructus)

Medicinal Dose: 3 grams daily as tea

Other Uses: Antiflatulent, diuretic, and mild antidiabetic

Caution: Herb may rarely cause photosensitivity; avoid herb if allergic to celery; avoid large amounts of herb.

Dandelion (Taraxaci herba)

Medicinal Dose: 5 grams in capsule form or as tincture or tea three times a day

Other Uses: Antidiabetic and diuretic

Caution: Dandelion may rarely cause contact dermatitis; patients with bile duct blockage, gall bladder problems, or bowel obstruction should not use.

Dill (Anethi fructus)

Medicinal Dose: 3 grams daily as tincture or tea

Other Uses: Antiflatulent and diuretic

Caution: None.

Hops (Lupuli strobulus)

Medicinal Dose: 500 mg of dry extract daily; one to two cups of tea daily; one bottle of beer daily

Other Uses: For anxiety and insomnia

Caution: None, but do not use hops if depressed.

Marshmallow Root (Althaeae radix)

Medicinal Dose: Two (2) 500 mg capsules three times a day; 60 grams daily as tincture or tea

Other Uses: Diuretic

Caution: Marshmallow root rarely may cause allergic reaction.

Oat Straw, Oats (Avenae stramentum)

Medicinal Dose: 100 grams daily

Other Uses: Diuretic and for anxiety and depression

Caution: Do not use if patient has celiac disease.

Quinoa (Chenopodium quinoa)

Medicinal Dose: 45 grams daily

Other Uses: For constipation, diabetes, hypertension, and high cholesterol; as an antioxidant

Caution: Risks are minimal provided leaves are not eaten in excess (contain oxalic acid).

Red Raspberry (Rubi idaei folium)

Medicinal Dose: 2.7 grams as three (3) 300 mg capsules three times a day, or daily as tincture or tea

Other Uses: Nutritive

Caution: Red raspberry rarely may cause loose stools and/or nausea; may decrease milk supply if used for greater than two weeks.

Red Clover (Trifolium pretense)

Medicinal Dose: 40 mg to 80 mg daily as tincture or tea

Other Uses: For estrogenic properties and as expectorant

Caution: Do not exceed recommended dosage; avoid fermented Red Clover; patients taking anticoagulants and/or aspirin should not use (contains coumarin, a blood thinner).

Stinging Nettle (Urtica dioica and Urtica urens)

Medicinal Dose: 1.8 grams as one (1) 600 mg capsule three times a day, or one cup of tea two to three times a day; 2 ½ mL to 5 mL of tincture three times a day

Other Uses: Mild diuretic and for mild gastrointestinal upset

Caution: Stinging nettle may cause mild diuresis and/or mild gastrointestinal upset.

Vervain (Verbena officinalis)

Medicinal Dose: 30 grams to 50 grams leaves daily as tea

Use: For anxiety and hypertension

Caution: Do not use if pregnant due to oxytocic (uterine stimulant) properties.

Summary

Nursing women who use herbals should use the same diligence and cautions as when using Food and Drug Administration (FDA) regulated drugs. The fact that many manufacturers promote their products as "natural" does not always imply that using them is usually safe. Unlike the regulation of prescription and OTC medicines, the FDA does not regulate herbal products in the same manner. At one time, the FDA regulated herbals under food manufacturing regulations. As of October 1994, under new FDA regulatory requirements, firms are responsible for determining that dietary supplements, including herbals, are safe and that any representations or claims made are substantiated by adequate evidence that they are not false or misleading. Please note that herbals purchased as food products continue to be regulated by the FDA under food regulations. Herbal products are required to be free of contaminants. Herbal labels may not make unfounded health and medical claims. Because of this situation, active ingredients may be present in more or less amounts than the herbal package label lists. Unknown harmful ingredients may potentially be present. Strengths of herbal product ingredients may vary depending upon the particular plant used, the part of the plant used, and where, when, and how the herb was processed. These inconsistencies can lead to differences in effectiveness and potentially harmful adverse effects in the mother and/or her nursling. Consumers, especially breastfeeding mothers, should purchase herbals from reputable manufacturers and from pharmacies where they can consult with knowledgeable pharmacists on proper use (PDR, 2011).

These herbals can be found in many recipes. This allows breastfeeding mothers to potentially enhance their milk supply while eating healthy, tasty, and necessary foods. By using the plant or seeds in recipes, the mother knows what herb she is eating and the amount she is ingesting. If possible, buy and use fresh herbs and spices. Look for bright colors and invigorating aromas for any dried herbs or seeds. Buying herbs and spices in the bulk sections of grocery, health, or ethnic stores allows you to see and smell first.

For mothers who are having serious problems with milk supply, I strongly encourage you to work with a certified lactation consultant. An excellent reference book is *The Nursing Mother's Herbal* by Sheila Humphrey. This book contains extensive information on galactogogue herbs and how to use them.

Recipes

Many of my lactation consultant friends have encouraged me over the years to publish a galactogogue recipe book. Many copyright-free recipes that contain galactogogues are available. I have compiled over 225 (including sub-recipes) of these recipes and categorized them by galactogogue ingredients. Many contain more than one galactogogue that make the recipes an added bonus. As you will notice, included are ethnic recipes that have been used by cultures over many years, often for their milk production effects.

I have tried to include a wide variety of beverages, breads, soups, salads, entrees, and desserts to provide a constant galactogogue source of menu items for eating and drinking while breastfeeding. I have put the galactogogues in **bold** letters whenever they appear in a recipe. Major and minor galactogogues are capitalized. Miscellaneous galactogogues are bolded and begin with small letters. Some recipes have more than one galactogogue.

For all recipes, I have standardized the terminology and units of measurement used. Note: Tablespoon is abbreviated as tbsp and teaspoon is abbreviated as tsp in the recipes.

I have included sub-recipes to limit having to look these up. I have eliminated any anti-galactogogue ingredients in the recipes and modified directions for consistency to ensure making (compounding) the recipes easier. The reader can decide upon the amount of each they wish to make.

Some of the recipes are flavored with alcoholic beverages. The small amount used is not likely to impact breastfeeding - most or all of the alcohol will evaporate during the cooking process. Although the liquor gives the dish a distinctive flavor, if you or your baby are sensitive to alcohol, leave out this ingredient.

Unless otherwise indicated below the recipe name, the recipes were found on the website CookEatShare.com. Many were modified when taste-tested.

My pharmacy and cooking background has greatly influenced the presentation of these galactogogue recipes. I continue to compound and cook to my thorough enjoyment as I counsel mothers and healthcare professionals on the use of medications and herbals during breastfeeding.

Enjoy your breastfeeding and enjoy all you eat while breastfeeding.

Bon appétit!

Cham masit sum nee dah!

Smacznego!

Alfalfa

It is interesting in that people who are allergic to peanuts or legumes may also be allergic to **Alfalfa**.

Alfalfa (Medicago sativa)

Type: Minor galactogogue

Medicinal Dose: Up to 60 grams daily (one to two capsules four times a day)

Other Uses: Diuretic and laxative

Caution: Alfalfa may cause loose stools and/or photosensitivity; do not use if allergic to peanuts and/or legumes; do not use in patients with systemic lupus erythematosus (SLE).

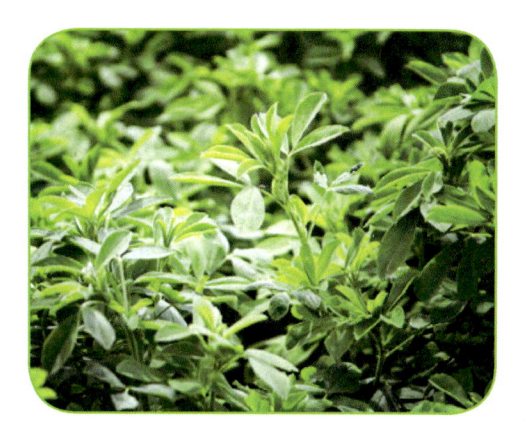

Appetizers

Deviled Eggs

(24 Deviled Eggs)

1 tbsp salt

12 large eggs

1 (19-ounce) can **chickpeas** (garbanzo beans), rinsed and drained

1 tbsp curry powder

3 tbsp yogurt (or more, if necessary)

2 tbsp lemon juice

½ tsp Tabasco sauce (or more or less, to taste)

1 tbsp paprika

½ cup **Alfalfa** leaves, finely chopped, as garnish

Bring large pot of water to a boil. Add salt. Gently drop in eggs. Cook for 12 minutes. Drain. Place in cold water. Crack and peel.

Cut eggs in half lengthwise. Remove yolks. Place egg whites, hole side up, on serving dish.

In a food processor, puree **chickpeas**, curry, yogurt, lemon juice, cooked egg yolks, and Tabasco sauce until very smooth. Taste and adjust seasoning.

Pipe (using a conical cone) or spoon filling into egg white holes.

Top with a dash of paprika and a sprinkle of chopped **alfalfa** leaves.

Breads

Vegetable Pizza Bread

(8 servings)

2 packages crescent rolls

2 (8 oz) packages cream cheese, softened

¾ cup salad dressing of your choice

1 tsp **Garlic** powder

1 tsp celery seeds

½ tsp **Dill** seeds

2 cups **Alfalfa** leaves, chopped

1 cup tomatoes, minced

½ cup green onions, chopped

½ cup green peppers, chopped

½ cup **mushrooms**, minced

1 **carrot**, shredded

1 cup **sunflower seeds**

2 cups cheddar cheese, grated

Unroll crescent rolls and place flat on a lightly greased cookie sheets to form mini pizza crusts. Do not let pizza crusts touch each other. Bake according to package directions to light brown color. Let cool.

Mix cream cheese, salad dressing, **Garlic** powder, celery seeds, and **Dill** seeds. Spread ⅛ of mixture over top of each pizza crust.

Mix **Alfalfa**, tomatoes, green onions, green peppers, **mushrooms**, and **carrot** together. Spread ⅛ of mixture over top of each pizza.

Sprinkle each pizza with **sunflower seeds** and grated cheese.

Chill for several hours.

Serve cool.

Salads

Asian Noodle Salad

(4 servings; Korean Ancestors' recipe)

1 pound linguine

1 red bell pepper, chopped

1 yellow bell pepper, chopped

1¼ cups bok choy, chopped

⅓ cup **carrots**, diced

1 cup celery, diced

4 **mushrooms**, thinly sliced

12 pea pods, cut diagonally into pieces

1 cup **Alfalfa** leaves, chopped

¼ cup sesame oil

¼ cup vegetable oil

2 tbsp soy sauce

¾ tsp orange marmalade

¾ tsp honey

½ tsp salt

1 tsp ground black pepper

In a large pot of salted boiling water, cook linguine according to package directions. When pasta is firm, but NOT hard, drain and set aside.

In the pasta pot, combine all other ingredients.

Pour pasta back into pot, and stir thoroughly until all ingredients are mixed together evenly and thoroughly.

Place pasta salad in a large bowl, cover, and refrigerate at least a few hours or overnight (even better) before serving.

Avocado Shrimp

(4 servings)

1 cup **Alfalfa** leaves

16 cherry tomatoes, halved

2 cups **lettuce**, shredded

2 soft avocados, peeled, halved, and seeds removed

2 cups cooked shrimp, shelled and deveined

1 lemon, cut in half

French dressing, as needed

Arrange ¼ cup **Alfalfa** leaves and 8 cherry tomato halves around the perimeter of each of 4 salad plates.

In the center of each salad plate, put ½ cup shredded **lettuce**.

Place an avocado half on bed of shredded **lettuce** on each plate. Using half of the lemon, squeeze a little lemon juice on each avocado.

Spoon ½ cup shrimp into cavity of each avocado.

Slice other half of lemon and use as garnish on each plate.

Top with French dressing.

Tossed Salad

(4 servings; Nice family recipe)

Salad

- 3 cups **spinach**, torn
- 3 cups iceberg **lettuce**, torn
- 1 (16-ounce) can **green beans**, drained and chilled
- 12 cherry tomatoes, halved
- 1 cup **Alfalfa** leaves, chopped
- ⅓ cup chestnuts, drained
- 1 small onion, sliced and pushed into rings
- 6 slices bacon, fried and crumbled
- 6 hard boiled eggs, chopped

Herb Dressing

- ¾ cup olive oil
- ¼ cup red wine vinegar
- 1 tsp sugar
- 1 tbsp **Garlic**, peeled and chopped or minced
- ½ tsp dry mustard
- ¼ tsp oregano
- ⅛ tsp ground black pepper

In a large bowl, combine all salad ingredients, except bacon and eggs.
In a small bowl, combine all herb-dressing ingredients with a whisk.
Top salad with bacon and eggs.
Serve with herb dressing.

Soups

Red Borscht Soup

(4 servings; Polish ancestors' recipe)

1 medium **beet**, scrubbed and cut into chunks

1 medium **carrot**, sliced

1 medium cucumber, cut into chunks

1 medium green bell pepper, seeded and coarsely minced

1 lemon, peeled, halved, and seeds removed

1 ripe avocado, peeled, seeds removed, and quartered

½ cup **spinach** leaves, packed

½ cup **Alfalfa** sprouts, packed

½ cup fresh **Dill**, minced

2 tbsp Bragg Liquid Aminos (or cider vinegar)

⅛ tsp freshly ground black pepper

2 cups vegetable stock (or vegetable bouillon)

1 cup **Alfalfa** leaves, chopped, plus as garnish

In a food processor fitted with the "S" blade, pulse **beet**, **carrot**, cucumber, bell pepper, and lemon until finely minced.

Add avocado, **spinach**, **Alfalfa** sprouts, **Dill**, liquid Aminos (or cider vinegar), and pepper.

With food processor running, gradually add vegetable stock and process until smooth.

Transfer soup to a bowl, cover, and chill at least 2 hours.

Serve soup in individual bowls, garnishing each with **Alfalfa** leaves.

Entrees

California Chicken Roll

(2 servings)

1 avocado, thinly sliced

½ cup **lettuce**, shredded

1 small tomato, diced

1 (5-ounce) chicken breast, cooked and cut into ½ inch cubes

1 ounce bacon bits

3 thin slices Swiss cheese, cut into small squares

½ tsp **basil**

½ tbsp **Garlic**, minced

½ cup mayonnaise

2 (10-inch) flour tortilla

½ cup **Alfalfa** leaves, chopped

Chop all but 6 slices of the avocado. Mix chopped avocado with **lettuce**, tomato, chicken, bacon bits, and Swiss cheese.

Add **basil** and **garlic** to mayonnaise and mix well.

Spread mayonnaise mixture on one side of each tortilla. At one end of each tortilla, spread ½ of the salad mixture. Place 3 slices of avocado on top of salad mixture and sprinkle with ¼ cup **Alfalfa** leaves. Roll each tortilla tightly and cut in half.

Serve.

Chicken Tacos

(4 servings)

4 cups **chicken broth**

1½ chicken breasts, skinned and deboned

4 (10-inch) flour tortillas

2 ripe tomatoes, diced

½ white onion, diced

½ head leaf **lettuce**, shredded

½ cup **Alfalfa** leaves, chopped

½ cup cheddar cheese, grated

½ cup tomato salsa

In a medium saucepan, bring broth to a boil. Add chicken. Reduce heat to medium-high and cook 20-25 minutes or until chicken is tender. Cool. Shred chicken.

Steam tortillas in a steamer basket or in a microwave covered with a moist paper towel until warm and soft.

Fill center of each tortilla with ½ of the chicken, tomatoes, onions, **lettuce**, **Alfalfa** leaves, and cheese. Top with salsa. Fold tortilla in half to make a taco.

Serve.

Korean Cold Spicy Noodles (Bibum Myun)

(2 servings; Korean ancestors' recipe)

2 servings soba (buckwheat) noodles

1 tbsp red pepper paste (gochujang) (divided) (available at Korean and Asian markets)

½ cucumber, thinly sliced

½ cup kimchi (available at Korean and Asian markets), thinly sliced

2-3 pieces red leaf **lettuce**, thinly shredded

2 hard-boiled eggs, sliced

½ tsp **sesame seeds** (garnish)

1-2 cups **Alfalfa** leaves, chopped, as garnish

Boil noodles for approximately 7 minutes or until noodles separate on their own (best to have slightly undercooked noodles as opposed to overcooked noodles, as they will continue to soften as eaten). For extra spiciness, add red pepper paste to noodles as they cook. Drain noodles under cold water for several minutes. Set aside.

Prepare cucumber and kimchi by thinly slicing into 2-inch strips.

Shred **lettuce** and lay in a bowl as a bed for noodles.

Place cooled noodles on top of bed of **lettuce**.

Top with sliced cucumbers, kimchi, and eggs.

Garnish with **sesame seeds** and **Alfalfa** leaves.

Serve with additional red pepper paste.

Roast Beef Sandwich

(4 servings)

⅓ cup low-fat sour cream

2 tbsp Dijon mustard

2 tsp prepared horseradish

4 individual French loaves

4 slices provolone cheese, cut in half

1 pound thinly sliced cooked roast beef

1 cup **Alfalfa** leaves, chopped

Preheat oven to 350 degrees.

Combine sour cream, mustard, and horseradish.

Split French loaves in half horizontally.

Spread ¼ of the sour cream mixture on top and bottom side of each French bread loaf. On the bottom side of each loaf, put 1 slice of cheese and ¼ of the roast beef. Top with French bread top.

Wrap the sandwich in aluminum foil and bake for 25 minutes.

Remove from oven, put ¼ cup of **Alfalfa** leaves on top of roast beef on each sandwich, and replace bread tops.

Cut each sandwich in half and serve.

Shrimp Sandwich

(4 servings)

4 tbsp fresh **Ginger** root, peeled and chopped

1⅓ cups mayonnaise

6 tbsp Dijon mustard

8 slices rye bread, toasted lightly

20 radishes, trimmed and sliced thin

2 cups **Alfalfa** leaves, chopped and lightly packed

1½ pounds small shrimp, cooked your favorite way – broiled, grilled, boiled, or fried

4 tsp lemon juice

In a small bowl, stir together **Ginger** root, mayonnaise, and mustard.

Spread 1 tbsp of **Ginger** mayonnaise on each piece of rye toast. Arrange radishes, **Alfalfa** leaves, and shrimp decoratively on toast.

Stir lemon juice into remaining mayonnaise. Drizzle over top.

Serve.

Smoked Turkey Asparagus Melt

(1 serving)

5 slices smoked turkey, thinly sliced
5 pieces fresh **asparagus**, blanched until tender
2 pieces wheat or rye bread
Butter, as spread
Thousand Island dressing, as spread
2 pieces Monterey Jack cheese, ⅛-inch thick
¾ cup **Alfalfa** leaves, chopped

Roll one turkey slice around each piece of **asparagus**.

Brush each slice of bread with butter on one side and Thousand Island dressing on other side. Place in nonstick skillet or grill, dressing side up.

On one slice of bread, place cheese. On other slice of bread, place turkey rolls in single layer.

Grill bread until bread is golden brown and cheese starts to melt.

Remove from pan and place **Alfalfa** leaves on top of turkey rolls.

Place slice of bread with melted cheese on top of bread with turkey rolls. Cut in half.

Serve.

Tuna Burgers

(4 servings; Nice family recipe)

2 large eggs
⅓ cup dry breadcrumbs
1 tbsp fresh **Dill**, minced
1 tbsp prepared horseradish
2 tsp Dijon mustard
¼ tsp ground black pepper
1 pinch salt
1 (13-ounce) can water-packed tuna, drained
2 green onions, chopped

1 celery stalk, minced

1 tbsp vegetable oil

4 whole wheat hamburger buns

1-2 cups **Alfalfa** leaves, chopped, as garnish

In bowl, lightly beat eggs. Fold in bread crumbs, **Dill**, horseradish, mustard, pepper, and salt. Add tuna, onions, and celery, and mix well. Shape into four ½-inch thick patties.

In nonstick skillet, heat oil over medium heat. Cook patties, turning once, for 10 minutes, until golden and set.

Place patties in buns.

Garnish with **Alfalfa** leaves.

Veggie Burgers

(4 servings)

2½ cups canned **chickpeas** (garbanzo beans), drained and rinsed

4 large eggs

1 tsp salt

1 tbsp **Coriander seeds**

1 onion, finely diced

Zest (colored portion of peel) of 1 large lemon, grated

1 cup **Alfalfa** leaves, chopped

1 cup whole-grain bread crumbs, toasted

1 tbsp extra-virgin olive oil

½ teaspoon freshly ground black pepper

Hamburger buns

1 tomato, sliced (optional)

1 cup onions, sliced and sautéed (optional)

1 cup **mushrooms**, sliced and sautéed (optional)

1 avocado, sliced (optional)

Combine **chickpeas**, eggs, and salt in a food processor. Puree until mixture is the consistency of hummus.

Pour into mixing bowl. Stir in **Coriander seeds**, onion, lemon zest, and

Alfalfa leaves. Add breadcrumbs. Let sit for a few minutes.

Form into 12 (1½-inch-thick) patties. The mixture may seem too moist to form into patties, but they will harden like a pancake. The moistness makes for a nicely textured burger.

Heat oil in a heavy skillet over medium-low heat, add four patties, cover, and cook for 7-10 minutes, until bottoms begin to brown (check after 3-4 minutes for color and turn down heat if browning too much). Turn up heat if there is no browning after 10 minutes.

Flip patties and cook for 7 minutes, or until golden.

Remove from skillet and cool on a wire rack.

Cook remaining patties.

Serve on hamburger buns with any or all of the optional toppings.

Anise

A**nise** has a licorice taste that makes cookies and pizzelles a very special Christmas and holiday treat.

Anise (Anisi fructus)

Type: Minor galactogogue

Medicinal Dose: 3.5 grams to 7 grams as tincture or tea, 5 to 6 times a day

Other Uses: For anxiety and as antiflatulent

Caution: Anise may cause an allergic reaction.

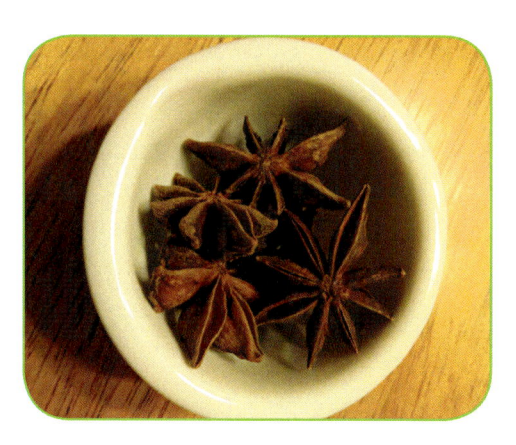

Salads

Crab Salad

(12 servings; Maine lobsterman recipe)

3 pounds fresh lump crab

⅓ cup fresh **Anise** (or fresh **Fennel**), minced

⅓ cup celery, minced

¼ cup shallot, minced

¼ cup red bell pepper, minced

1½ tsp orange zest (colored portion of peel), grated

1 tbsp chives, chopped

1 orange, juiced

½ lemon

½ cup extra-virgin olive oil

Salt, to taste

Ground black pepper, to taste

1 pound **lettuce**

4 fresh avocadoes, finely chopped

Mix all ingredients, except **lettuce** and avocadoes. Refrigerate for at least 1 hour.

Spread crab mixture on a sheet pan. Heat in a 450 degree oven, approximately 3-5 minutes.

While crab mixture is warming, arrange **lettuce** on 12 plates.

Spoon approximately 2 - 2½ ounces warmed crab mixture over **lettuce** on each plate. Top with chopped avocado.

Serve.

Entrees

Anise Turkey Curry

(2 servings)

2 star **Anise**, whole pieces, not broken (available in Asian markets)

1 tbsp grated **Ginger**

1 tsp **turmeric** powder

½ tsp cayenne pepper

1 tsp **Garlic** salt

1 tbsp honey

8 ounces turkey breast, chopped

2 tbsp red onion, chopped

½ cup matchstick **carrots**

2 ounces hot **chicken stock**

2 spring onions, chopped

½ cup baby corn, chopped

½ cup **spinach**

Vegetable oil, for frying

Steamed **rice** (or boiled, chopped potatoes)

Crush the star **Anise** with **Ginger**, **turmeric**, cayenne pepper, and **Garlic** salt. Mix in honey.

Coat turkey with mixture and let marinate for 15 minutes.

Heat oil in a wok or skillet. Add turkey and cook until brown. Add **carrots** and cook until tender. Add red onion and cook until translucent.

Add **chicken stock**, then turn down to simmer.

Add spring onions and baby corn. Continue to simmer for 5 minutes.

Stir in **spinach** until it wilts.

Serve over steamed **rice** or boiled, chopped potatoes.

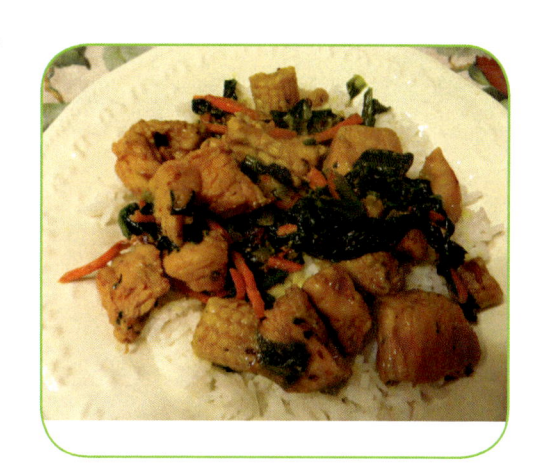

BBQ Sichuan Pork Ribs

(8 servings)

3 **Garlic** cloves, crushed

1 (2-inch) piece fresh **Ginger**, grated

2 tsp Sichuan peppercorns, finely crushed

½ tsp ground black pepper

1 tsp star **Anise**, finely ground

1 tsp Chinese five spice powder

6 tbsp dark soy sauce

3 tbsp sunflower oil

1 tbsp sesame oil

4 baby back pork rib slabs or spare ribs

Note: Exotic spices can be found in Asian markets, gourmet markets, or on-line.

Mix together **Garlic**, **ginger**, Sichuan peppercorns, pepper, star **Anise**, Chinese five spice powder, soy sauce, sunflower oil, and sesame oil.

Marinate ribs in spice mixture overnight.

Remove ribs from refrigerator 1 hour before cooking and bring to room temperature. Pat dry.

Pour marinade into a pan and bring to a boil; then lower heat and simmer for 3 minutes.

Place ribs on rack in indirect heat on grill that is 250-300 degrees. Turn every 30 minutes until done. Ribs are done when rack is lifted in the middle a bit, and threatens to split in two. Baby back ribs will take approximately 90 minutes/spare ribs will take approximately 150 minutes.

After the ribs are done, baste one side with marinade and cook 3 minutes; turn and repeat with other side. Repeat again so each side gets basted twice.

Braised Beef Short Ribs with Anise and Ginger

(6 servings)

⅓ cup soy sauce

⅓ cup dry sherry (or wine or dry vermouth)

2 tbsp light brown sugar, packed

1 (14-ounce) can diced tomatoes

½ cup water

2 star **Anise**, whole pieces, not broken (available in Asian markets)

3 pounds beef short ribs on the bone, cut into 3-inch lengths

Salt, to taste

Freshly ground black pepper, to taste

1½ tbsp vegetable oil plus more, if needed

4 **Garlic** cloves, crushed and peeled

3 small leeks, cut in half and then into 1-inch pieces

1 (1-inch) piece fresh **Ginger**, approximately diameter of a quarter, cut into 8 slices

2 tbsp scallions, thinly sliced and cut on the diagonal, for garnish

Set rack in middle level of oven and preheat oven to 325 degrees.

Mix together soy sauce, sherry (or wine or vermouth), brown sugar, tomatoes, water, and star **Anise** in a bowl. Set aside.

Dry ribs and season lightly with salt and generously with pepper.

Brown ribs in batches in a heavy, ovenproof pot. Remove as browned, adding more oil, if necessary.

When all ribs are browned, pour off fat (if any) from casserole and reduce heat to low. Add **garlic**, leeks, and **Ginger**. Cook for one minute.

Return ribs to pot. Pour soy sauce mixture over them. Bring liquid to a simmer and cover.

Transfer pot to oven and cook for approximately 2-2½ hours or until ribs are tender when pierced with a fork. Turn ribs occasionally while they are cooking. If liquid gets low, add a little water.

Transfer ribs to a serving platter.

Discard **Ginger** and star **Anise** from braising liquid. Remove grease, then pour over ribs.

Serve hot garnished with thinly sliced scallions.

Note: Ribs are best when made a day or two before serving.

Cheesy Anise Chicken

(4 servings)

2 tbsp soy sauce
1 tbsp honey
2 tsp star **Anise**, ground (divided)
8 ounces chicken thighs, deboned and chopped
Vegetable oil, for frying
1 (14½-ounce) can diced tomatoes
4 ounces sweet corn
4 ounces plum tomatoes, halved
4 ounces **mushrooms**, sliced
2 tbsp red onion, chopped
4 ounces grated cheese

Mix soy sauce, honey, and 1 tsp **Anise**. Pour over chicken in a bowl. Let marinate for 15 minutes.

Heat oil in a pan. Brown onion and chicken.

Add diced tomatoes, corn, plum tomatoes, **mushrooms**, and onion, plus remaining 1 tsp **anise**, tossing well. Heat vegetables through.

Remove from heat and stir in cheese.

Serve with steamed **rice**.

Chinese Braised Oxtails with Root Vegetables

(8 servings; Korean ancestors' recipe)

2 tbsp soy sauce
1 tbsp water
1 tbsp **rice** wine (double distilled is preferred; can substitute Sake)
1 tsp brown sugar
4 tbsp canola oil
6 (¼-inch) thick, fresh **Ginger** (divided)
5-6 stalks green onion, cut ¼-inch thick (save 2 tbsp for garnish)
8 large **Garlic** cloves, peeled and flattened slightly

1 tbsp Chinese ground bean sauce

12 (2-2½-inch thick) oxtail pieces (approximately 4½ pounds), fat trimmed

2 cups low-salt **chicken broth**

½ cup soy sauce

8 star **Anise**, whole pieces, not broken (available in Asian markets)

3 tbsp dark brown sugar

20 Chinese dry **mushroom** or shitake **mushroom**, soaked in water for approximately 2 hours, until softened

3 Chinese radishes, cut in ½-inch slices

3 **carrots**, cut in ½-inch slices

Mix soy sauce, water, **rice** wine, and sugar for sauce before cooking.

To brown oxtails, heat oil over medium heat in a wok or Dutch oven. When slight smoke appears, add 2 slices of **Ginger**, 2 tbsp green onions, 3 **Garlic** cloves, and ground bean sauce. Stir and cook for 20-30 seconds.

Add oxtails and sauce to wok. Brown oxtails slightly on all sides, approximately 5-8 minutes.

Transfer oxtails to Dutch oven. Add **chicken stock**, green onions, soy sauce, **Garlic**, star **Anise**, **Ginger**, and brown sugar.

Add enough water to cover oxtails by ½ inch; bring to a boil. Reduce heat to low, partially cover, and simmer until very tender, adding more water by ½ cupfuls as needed to keep oxtails covered. Cooking time is approximately 3 hours.

Approximately 2 hours into cooking, add **mushrooms**, Chinese radishes, and **carrots**. Add water, if needed, to keep vegetables covered. Cook until vegetables are softened.

To serve, garnish with green parts of green onion.

Oriental Chicken

(4 servings; Korean ancestors recipe)

4 plump chicken thighs, skin removed

5 ounces Chinese brown **rice** wine

3 ounces soy sauce

1 heaping tsp fresh **Ginger**, peeled and grated

4 **Garlic** cloves, crushed

5 star **Anise**, whole pieces, not broken (available in Asian markets)

1 tsp sesame oil

2 ounces water

4 bowls cooked **rice** (sticky white, Korean style)

1 small red chili, deseeded and cut into fine shreds

1 spring onion, cut into fine shreds

Preheat oven to 400 degrees.

Place skinned chicken thighs in a casserole dish (one that can go from stove to oven). Mix **rice** wine, soy sauce, **Ginger**, **Garlic**, **Anise**, and sesame oil with water in a bowl. Pour over chicken.

Place casserole over medium heat on stove and bring liquid to a boil.

Transfer to preheated oven (no need to cover) and bake on center shelf for 30 minutes, turning chicken halfway through the cooking time.

Serve cooked chicken on a bed of **rice**. Pour cooking sauce over chicken and **rice**. Garnish with shreds of chili and spring onion sprinkled on top.

Smoked Pork Loin

(4 servings)

1 (2-pound) boneless pork loin

2 quarts water

6 ounces salt

2 ounces brown sugar

1 cup apple cider

1 apple, chopped

2 cinnamon sticks, whole

2 star **Anise**, whole pieces, not broken (available in Asian markets)

1 tbsp **Fennel** seed

Place pork in ceramic dish or glass bowl.

Mix rest of ingredients in another bowl. Stir until sugar and salt are dissolved. Pour over pork. Refrigerate for 24-36 hours.

Remove from liquid and dry pork loin.

Roast in 350 degree oven or on barbecue grill until internal temperature reaches 145 degrees.

Let rest.

Slice and serve.

Tuna Noodle Casserole

(4 servings)

4 servings ramen noodles

1 tbsp soy sauce

1 star **Anise**, whole piece, not broken (available in Asian markets)

1 tsp peppercorns

½ tsp whole cloves

1 tsp **Fennel** seeds

1 (1-inch) fresh **Ginger** root, peeled and finely chopped

1 tbsp olive oil

1 tuna steak

In a pot, bring water to boil. Add noodles. Boil for 2 minutes. Drain noodles; cover with soy sauce.

Using a mortar and pestle or a grinder, grind star **Anise**, peppercorns, cloves, and **Fennel**. Add **Ginger** and olive oil and mix into a paste.

Coat the tuna with olive oil paste.

Heat pan. Sear tuna for 1 minute per side.

Slice tuna and place on top of noodles.

Sides

Zucchini with Anise

(4 servings)

2 tbsp olive oil

2 **Garlic** cloves, minced

1 tsp crushed red pepper flakes

2 medium zucchini, cut in 2-inch long matchsticks

1 tsp **Anise** seeds

1 tbsp fresh **basil**, minced

Salt, to taste

Ground black pepper, to taste

¼ cup grated Romano cheese

Sauté **Garlic** in oil until soft, but not browned.

Add pepper flakes and zucchini. Cook approximately 10 minutes, stirring occasionally.

Sprinkle in **Anise** seeds and cook for another minute. Remove from heat.

Add **basil**, and season with salt and pepper. Mix well.

Sprinkle with grated cheese and serve.

Desserts

Anise Cookies

(24 cookies; Nice family recipe)

2 cups flour

1 cup sugar

1 tsp baking soda

7 tbsp butter

3 egg yolks

1 lemon zest (colored portion of peel) and juice

1 tsp **Anise** seeds

Preheat oven to 350 degrees.

Sift together flour and baking soda into a medium bowl. Set aside.

Cream butter and sugar in a mixer. While on low speed, add eggs, lemon juice and zest, and **Anise** seeds. Slowly add dry ingredients and mix well.

Roll dough into small walnut size balls and press down.

Place formed cookies on parchment paper or a greased cookie sheet.

Bake for 10-12 minutes or until slightly golden.

Remove cookies from pan and place on a cooling rack.

Blueberry Biscotti

(24 biscotti)

3 tbsp unsalted butter, softened

10 tbsp sugar

1½ cups flour, plus 2 tbsp flour for work surface

1 tsp baking powder

1 pinch salt

Zest (colored part of peel) of 1 lemon

2 large eggs

⅔ cup almond slivers

⅓ cup blueberries

1 tbsp **Anise** seeds

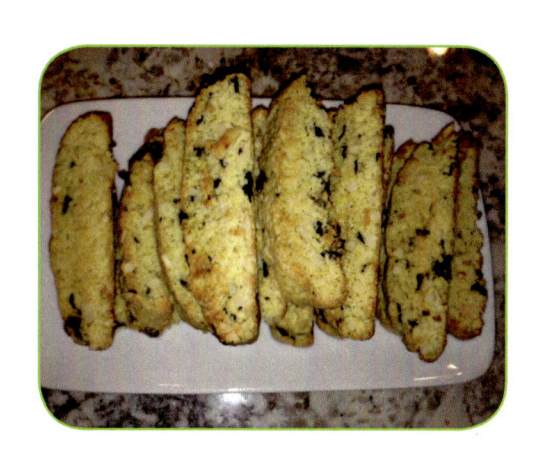

Preheat oven to 350 degrees. Line baking sheet with parchment paper.

Cream butter and sugar. Add flour, baking powder, salt, and lemon zest. Beat until just combined. Add eggs, one at a time, beating well after each addition.

Gently stir in almonds, blueberries, and **Anise** seeds.

On a lightly floured work surface, shape dough into a log – approximately 12 inches long.

Put log on parchment lined baking sheet. Flatten log, so it is approximately 4 inches wide and 1-2 inches tall. Bake for 35-40 minutes or until top is firm.

Allow log to cool for 10 minutes.

Cut log into ½-inch thick slices.

Place slices on lined baking sheet and bake 12-14 minutes or until golden brown and crisp.

Cool on wire rack.

Note: Biscotti can be stored in an airtight container in a cool, dry place up to two weeks.

Orange Anise Cake

(8 servings)

1 cup orange juice

1 tsp salt

3 large eggs, room temperature

1¼ cups milk

2 cups sugar

¼ cup orange liqueur, rum, brandy, or whisky (alcohol will evaporate during cooking)

1½ cups extra-virgin olive oil, plus more for oiling pans

1 tbsp grated lemon zest (colored potion of peel)

2 tsp **Anise** seeds

2 cups flour

½ tsp baking soda

½ tsp baking powder

6 tbsp lemon or orange marmalade (divided)

Preheat oven to 350 degrees. Prepare two 10-inch cake pans.

Reduce orange juice to ¼ cup over medium heat. Add salt, stir, and let cool.

Lightly beat eggs until frothy. Add milk, sugar, liqueur, olive oil, reduced orange juice, lemon zest, and **Anise** seeds. Mix for 1 minute until well blended.

Add flour, baking soda, and baking powder. Mix until well blended and smooth.

Pour half the mixture into each oiled cake pan. Bake for one hour.

Remove cakes from oven. While cakes are still warm, smear tops with 3 tbsp marmalade.

When cool, remove from pans and place one on top of the other on a cake plate.

Serve.

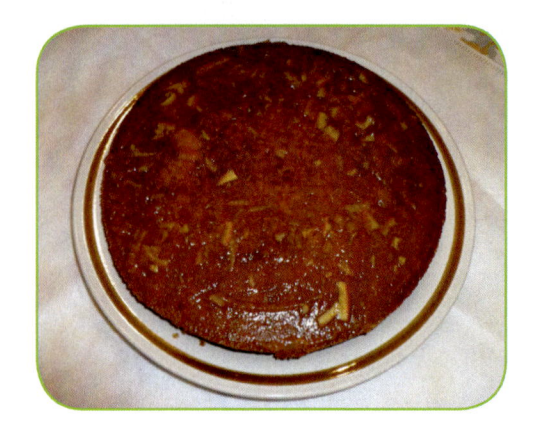

Pizzelles

(36 cookies; Nice family recipe)

3 eggs

¾ cup sugar

½ cup margarine, melted and cooled

4 tbsp **Anise** extract

1¾ cups flour

2 tsp baking powder

2 tbsp **Anise** and/or **Fennel** seeds

Water, as needed

Preheat pizzelle iron (available at retailers).

Cream together eggs and sugar; add margarine and **Anise** extract.

Add flour and baking powder, and mix until smooth.

Add **Anise** and/or **Fennel** seeds, and mix well.

If batter is too thick, add water, 1 tbsp at a time, until desired consistency.

Using a teaspoon, drop 1 spoonful of batter on the pizzelle iron for each cookie. (You can also put the batter in a Ziploc bag, snip off one small corner like a pastry bag, and squeeze out a teaspoon-sized dollop on the iron for each cookie. This gives better control, is much less sticky, and cleanup is easier.)

Beer (Barley/Hops)

Barley and **Hops** are two of the main ingredients in **Beer**. The use of alcohol during breastfeeding can be somewhat controversial. Some contraindicate the use of all alcohol while breastfeeding. Others say a little is okay. Alcohol evaporates when cooked, leaving only the flavor, which greatly enhances some recipes. However, if the breastfed infant is turned off by the smell or taste or if mom's milk supply is affected when alcohol is included in a recipe, then it would be prudent to avoid recipes containing **Beer**, wine, and other liquors.

Barley (Hordeum vulgare)

Type: Minor galactogogue

Medicinal Dose: 15 grams of **barley** extract; 1 to 2 cups of tea daily

Other Uses: For nutrition and aid to digestion

Caution: None.

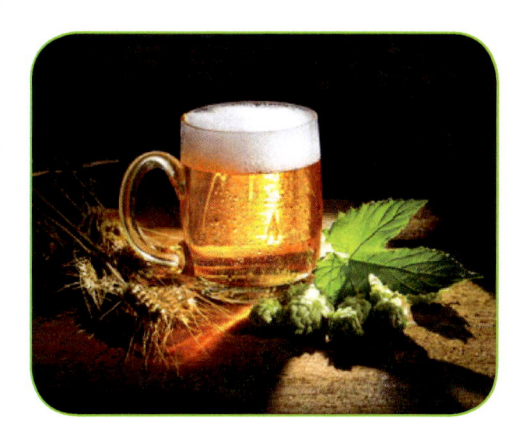

Hops (Lupuli strobulus)

Type: Minor galactogogue

Medicinal Dose: 500 mg of dry extract daily; 1 to 2 cups of tea daily

Other Uses: For anxiety and insomnia

Caution: None, but do not use **Hops** if depressed.

Appetizers

Beer Battered Onion Rings

(4 servings)

2 large onions

4 eggs (divided)

1 (12-ounce) can **Beer**

2 cups flour

1 tbsp salt

1 tbsp sugar

1 tbsp paprika (optional)

Preheat deep fryer.

Slice onions crosswise into approximately ¼ -½ inch thick slices. Punch out rings.

In a mixing bowl, whisk 2 eggs with **Beer**. Mix well. Whisk in flour, salt, sugar, and paprika (optional).

Separate the whites from the remaining 2 eggs. Whisk the 2 egg whites until fluffy.

Add half of the egg whites to mixing bowl with other ingredients. Fold in gently until blended. Add remaining egg whites.

Dip onion rings into batter, let drain slightly, and slowly place into deep fryer. Add rings until top of fryer is full. Gently turn rings as they brown. When golden brown, drain on paper towel to remove excess oil.

Repeat until all rings have been fried.

Serve with favorite dips.

Beer Battered Pickles

(4 servings)

Vegetable oil, for frying

1 egg

1 (12-ounce) can **Beer**

1 tbsp baking powder

2 cups flour
Salt, to taste
Ground black pepper, to taste
½ tsp mustard powder
½ tsp paprika
2 cups pickle chips
Ranch dipping sauce (recipe below)

Heat vegetable oil to 350 degrees in a fryer, heavy skillet, or Dutch oven.
Mix egg, **Beer**, baking powder, flour, and spices in a bowl.
Batter each pickle chip individually and fry until golden.
Serve with Ranch dipping sauce.

Ranch Dipping Sauce

½ cup mayonnaise
½ cup sour cream
¼ cup buttermilk
2 tbsp hot sauce (e.g., Frank's Red Hot)
1 tbsp apple cider vinegar
1 **Garlic** clove, minced
2 green onions, thinly sliced
Salt, to taste
Pepper, to taste

Mix all ingredients together in a bowl.
Serve with fried pickles.

Beer Cheese Spread

(Multiple servings)

1 pound extra sharp cheddar cheese, grated
½ cup **Beer**
1 tbsp Worcestershire sauce
2 tsp minced onion

½ tsp dry mustard

¼ tsp Tabasco sauce

Process all ingredients in a food processor.

Refrigerate overnight to allow flavors to blend.

Serve with flavored crackers.

Breads

Apple Cheddar Beer Bread

(1 loaf)

1 tbsp olive oil

½ cup shallots (or onion and/or chili peppers and/or herbs, to taste), finely chopped

½ cup gala apple, peeled and shredded

¼ tsp freshly black ground pepper

1 **Garlic** clove, minced

3 cups flour

3 tbsp sugar

2 tsp baking powder

1 tsp salt

1 cup smoked cheddar cheese (or similar cheese)

½ cup raisins

1 (12-ounce) can **Beer**

Cooking spray, as needed

2 tbsp butter, melted (divided)

Preheat oven to 375 degrees.

Sauté shallots and apple in oil until browned, stirring occasionally. Add pepper and **garlic**, cook another minute.

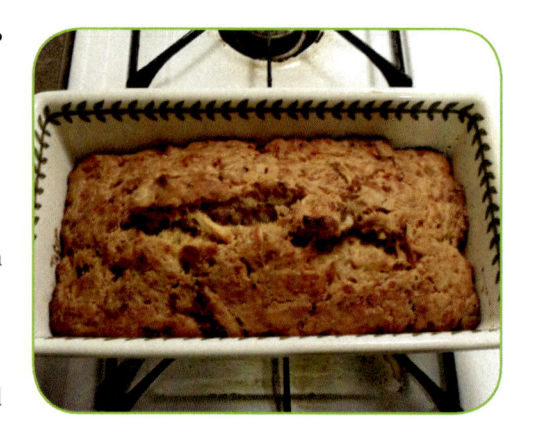

Combine flour, sugar, baking powder, and salt in a large bowl. Add onion/apple mixture, cheese, raisins, and **Beer**; stir until moist.

Pour batter into a prepared 9 by 5-inch loaf pan. Drizzle 1 tbsp of melted butter over batter and bake for 35-45 minutes.

Drizzle remaining butter over batter. Bake another 25 minutes or until bread is golden brown and a toothpick comes out clean. Cool.

Note: Flavors mellow out overnight. Bread may be better on second day.

Beer Bread

(1 loaf)

1 (12-ounce) can warm **Beer**

3 cups self-rising flour

3 tbsp sugar

1 tbsp butter, melted

Preheat oven to 350 degrees.

Combine **Beer**, flour, and sugar.

Pour into prepared bread pan and bake for 30 minutes or until golden brown.

Top with melted butter.

Condiments

Beer Bacon Spread

(Multiple servings)

1 (12-ounce) package smoked bacon, cut into 1 inch pieces

1 large onion, diced

4 **Garlic** cloves, minced

1 chili pepper, diced

1 tbsp marinade sauce

½ tsp paprika

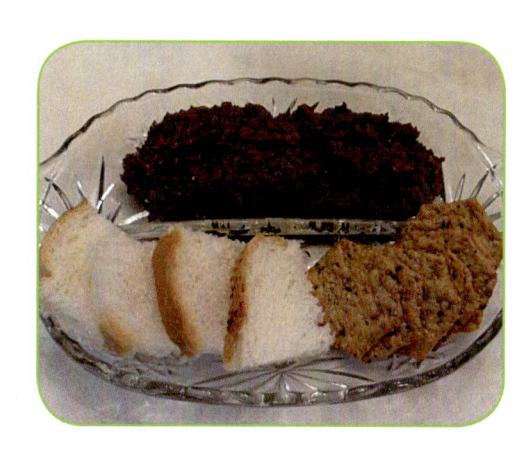

1 tbsp **molasses (black strap)**

1 cup brewed coffee

1 (12-ounce) can **Beer** (divided)

¼ cup maple syrup

Freshly ground black pepper, to taste

Fry bacon over medium heat until browned, but not crisp. Remove bacon.

Drain all but 1 tbsp of bacon grease from the pan. Fry onion and **Garlic** in the bacon grease until soft.

Add rest of ingredients and bring to a boil. Reduce heat and simmer uncovered for 2 hours. Add more **Beer** as needed to keep mixture from drying out.

Allow mixture to cool, then purée until smooth, with some texture.

Serve as spread on crackers or bread.

Soups

Beer Cheese Soup

(8 servings)

½ pound bacon, chopped

¾ cup onion, finely diced

½ cup celery, diced

¾ cup **carrots**, diced

1 tbsp **Garlic**, minced

1¼ cups flour

½ cup butter

4¾ cups **chicken stock**

2 (12-ounce) cans **Beer**

2 pounds Cheddar cheese, cut into chunks

3 cups heavy cream

1 tbsp dry mustard

Brown bacon. Drain on a paper towel. Remove bacon drippings, leaving about 1 tbsp in the pot.

Add onion, celery, **carrots**, and **garlic**, and sauté until soft.

Add flour and butter, stirring until flour is cooked.

Add **chicken stock** and **Beer**. Add half of the cooked bacon.

Using an immersion blender, blend until soup is smooth.

Bring soup to a boil. Reduce heat to low and gradually add cheese, cream, and mustard. Mix until smooth. Stir until added ingredients are warm.

Serve garnished with bacon.

Entrees

Beef Beer Chili

(8 servings)

1½ pounds beef sirloin tip roast, chuck roast, or top round roast, cut into 1/2-inch cubes

1½ pounds ground beef

¼ cup olive oil

3 medium onions, chopped

4 **Garlic** cloves, minced

3 jalapeño peppers, seeded and chopped

1 green bell pepper, seeded and chopped

1 tbsp ground **cumin**

¼ cup chili powder

1 tbsp paprika

1 (12-ounce) can **Beer**

1 (28-ounce) can chopped tomatoes

3 tbsp tomato paste

1 (14-ounce) can black beans

1 (4-ounce) can chopped green chilies

1 cup beef stock, as needed for desired consistency

Salt, to taste

Ground black pepper, to taste

Cornbread

Shredded cheese, optional

Coriander seeds, optional

Red onion, chopped, optional

Sour cream, optional

Heat oil in large, heavy pot.

Season beef cubes with salt and pepper. Brown in olive oil. When browned, remove from oil and drain. Add ground beef to pot and brown.

Add onions, **Garlic**, and peppers, and cook until onion is translucent.

Return beef cubes to pot. Stir in **cumin**, chili powder, and paprika, and cook 2-3 minutes.

Add **Beer**, stir well, and bring to a boil. Allow foam to subside, approximately 1 minute.

Add tomatoes and tomato paste; return to a boil. Add beef stock for desired consistency. Lower heat, cover, and simmer for 1½ hours or until beef cubes are fork tender, stirring occasionally.

Add beans and green chilies; cook another ½ hour. Season with salt and pepper, if desired.

Serve with cornbread and top with your choice of shredded cheese, **Coriander seeds**, red onion, and/or sour cream.

Beer Battered Prawns

(1-2 servings)

2 tbsp self-rising flour

¼ tsp paprika

½ tsp salt

½ tsp pepper

1 tbsp corn flour

1 egg

2 tsp vegetable oil

6 ounces cold **Beer**

10-12 medium prawns, cleaned and deveined

Vegetable oil, for deep-frying

Corn flour, for dusting

2 drops sesame oil

½ tsp cooking wine

1 dash salt

1 dash pepper

Mix self-rising flour, paprika, salt, pepper, and corn flour.

In a separate bowl, whisk eggs, oil, and **Beer**. Add flour mixture slowly and whisk into batter.

Make 2 slits in the back of each prawn. Dust each prawn with corn flour and coat with **Beer** batter.

Heat vegetable oil in wok or skillet until you see bubbles.

Fry prawns until golden brown. Drain.

Mix sesame oil, cooking wine, salt and pepper to make marinade.

Serve prawns with marinade.

Beer Brats

(6 servings)

2 tsp olive oil or butter (divided use)

6 bratwurst sausages

1 large sweet onion, sliced into ¼-inch rings

1 bell pepper, sliced into ¼ inch strips

6 ounces **Beer**

6 hotdog buns

Heat 1 tsp olive oil or butter in pan. Brown bratwurst sausages until deep golden brown. Remove from pan.

Add remaining 1 tsp olive oil or butter to drippings. Sauté onion rings and bell pepper until onions are limp and golden and pepper is soft.

Return bratwurst to pan and add **Beer**.

Cook over medium heat until **Beer** has formed a syrup, approximately 12-15 minutes.

Warm hotdog buns.

Place a bratwurst on each bun and top with onion/bell pepper syrup.

Serve.

Beer Grilled Pork Chops

(4 servings)

¼ cup soy sauce

2 tbsp brown sugar

2 tsp **Ginger** root, grated

1 cup **Beer**

4 bone-in pork chops, approximately ¾-inch thick

Mix soy sauce, brown sugar, **Ginger** root, and **Beer**.

Marinate pork chops in soy sauce mixture in refrigerator for 4-24 hours.

Remove pork chops from marinade and grill over medium-hot coals, turning once until pork chops reach desired doneness.

Serve.

Beer Marinated Pork Chops

(4 servings)

1 tbsp whole grain mustard (for a hotter mustard, add 1 tsp hot mustard)

2 **Garlic** cloves, crushed and chopped

½ cup tomato sauce (or ketchup)

1 (12-ounce) can **Beer**

⅓ cup Worcestershire sauce

1 tbsp loose brown sugar

4 large pork chops

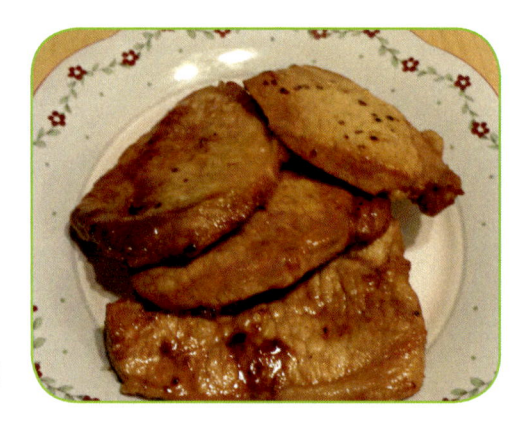

Mix together mustard, **garlic**, tomato sauce, **Beer**, Worcestershire sauce, and brown sugar.

Marinate pork chops in refrigerator overnight.

Remove from refrigerator approximately 2 hours before cooking.

Cook on grill or in oven. Cooking time will vary depending on thickness of pork chops and heat of coals or oven. Take care NOT to overcook because meat becomes chewy and loses much of its flavor.

Baste with marinade halfway through cooking process, then discard marinade. Do NOT baste with marinade when pork chops are nearly done.

Let pork chops rest approximately 5 minutes before serving.

Braised Beef Shank and Vegetables in Beer

(8 servings)

2-3 tbsp vegetable oil

4 pounds beef shanks

1 medium onion, chopped

4-5 bay leaves

1 bulb **Garlic**, separated into cloves and peeled

1 ripe medium tomato, chopped

2 celery stalks with leaves, chopped

2 **carrots**

1 (12-ounce) can **Beer**

1 pound small new potatoes (approximately 2 inches in diameter), well scrubbed

1 cup beef stock (optional)

Salt, to taste

Freshly cracked black pepper, to taste

Preheat oven to 375 degrees.

Heat oil in large ovenproof pot or casserole (with a lid) over medium-high heat; add beef shanks and brown on all sides. Remove pot from heat and remove shanks from pot.

Place onion, bay leaves, tomato, celery, **carrots**, and **Beer** in bottom of pot. Place beef shanks on top and season with salt and pepper. Cover and put in oven. Bake 2-3 hours, until meat is tender.

When meat is tender, add new potatoes and cook an additional 30 minutes or until potatoes are tender.

When done, remove beef shanks and potatoes from pot and place on a serving plate.

To make a sauce from the drippings and remaining vegetables, remove bay leaves and skim off fat. Puree using a hand held blender, regular blender,

Italian Style Beer Battered Seafood

(4 servings)

2 quarts vegetable cooking oil, for frying
1 cup flour plus flour for coating
2 tsp **Garlic** powder
½ tsp oregano
½ tsp **basil**
2 tbsp paprika
2 tsp salt
2 tsp ground black pepper
¼ tsp cayenne pepper
1 egg
1 (12-ounce) can **Beer**
2 pounds cod or haddock fillets, shrimp, scallops, and/or tilapia

Heat oil in a deep fat fryer to approximately 375 degrees.
Combine flour and spices. Add beaten egg and **Beer**. Mix well.
Coat seafood in flour, then dip in batter.
Fry in hot oil until browned and crispy. Drain on paper towels.
Serve with your favorite seafood sauce.

Sides

Spicy Rice with Beer

(3-4 servings)

½ cup onion, chopped
½ cup green bell pepper, chopped

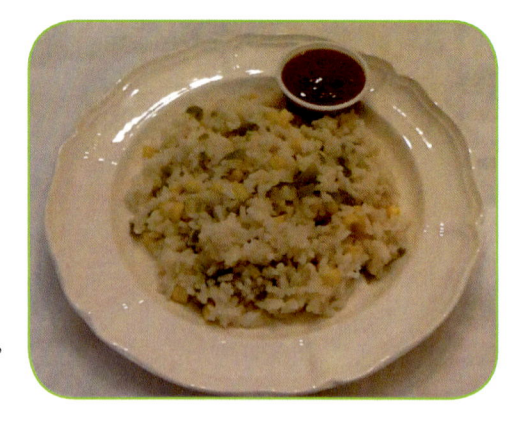

½ cup corn

1 tbsp butter

1 cup **chicken broth**

2 cups boiling water

1 cup uncooked long-grain **rice**

¾ cup **Beer**

¼ tsp salt

¼ tsp pepper

Picante sauce

Sauté onion, green bell pepper, and corn in butter until tender.

Add **chicken broth**.

Stir in **rice**, **Beer**, and seasonings, and bring to a boil.

Cover, reduce heat, and simmer 30 minutes or until liquid is absorbed and **rice** is tender.

Serve with Picante sauce.

Caraway

Being Polish, when I think of rye bread, the best rye bread contains **Caraway** seeds. **Caraway** seeds are also great with sauerkraut and cabbage.

Caraway (Carvi fructus)

Type: Minor galactogogue

Medicinal Dose: 1.5 grams to 6 grams daily as tincture, tea, or essential oil

Other Uses: For anxiety and as antiflatulent

Caution: Avoid large amounts of the essential oil form.

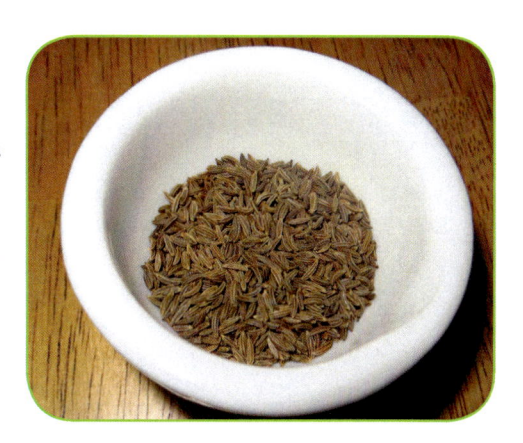

Breads

Caraway Cheese Muffins

(12 muffins)

1 cup corn meal

1 cup wheat flour

4 tsp baking powder

2 tsp sugar

1 tsp **Caraway** seeds, ground

1¼ tsp salt

¼ tsp ground pepper

1 cup Colby, Swiss, or cheddar cheese, coarsely grated

1 egg

1 cup milk

¼ cup butter, melted and cooled

1 tsp **Caraway** seeds, for sprinkling

Preheat oven to 350 degrees.

Process corn meal in food processor until consistency of flour.

Sift together processed corn meal, wheat flour, baking powder, sugar, **Caraway** seeds, salt, and pepper. Stir in cheese.

In another bowl, whisk together egg, milk, and butter. Add to flour mixture and stir batter until just combined.

Divide batter among 12 buttered muffin tins. Sprinkle with **Caraway** seeds.

Bake muffins for 25-30 minutes or until golden brown.

Let muffins cool a few minutes; then remove from tins.

Serve with soup or chili.

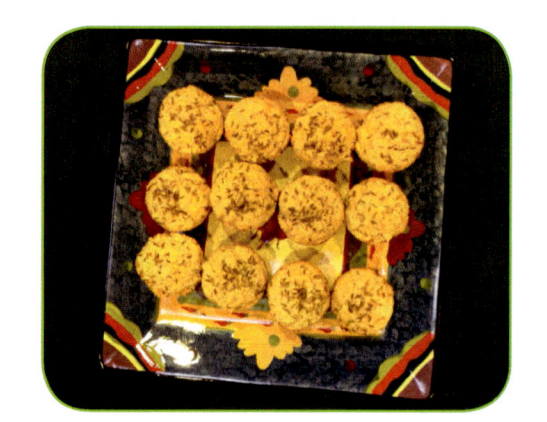

Sourdough Rye Bread (Rolls) with Caraway Seeds

(1 loaf; Polish ancestors' recipe)

Active Starter

2 cups warm water

1 package active dry yeast

2 cups flour

In a ceramic bowl, add warm water and yeast. Mix until yeast is dissolved.

Stir in flour and mix until smooth.

Pour into a plastic container that is at least 4 times larger than the starter, as starter will expand.

Cover plastic container with a cloth napkin held in place by a rubber band. Set starter in a warm place for five days.

Refrigerate and use starter as needed, at least once a week.

Feed starter daily with equal parts of water and flour, with 1 pinch salt.

Sourdough Bread

½ tbsp yeast

1 cup warm milk

2 tbsp brown sugar

1 cup active starter

2 tbsp butter, melted

½ cup rye flour

½ cup whole wheat flour

2 cups all purpose flour plus more, if needed

1 tsp salt

1 cup **Oatmeal** flakes, as topping

1 tbsp **molasses (black strap)**

1 tbsp **Caraway** seeds

In a large bowl, mix yeast with milk and brown sugar. Give a little stir and watch yeast foam.

Add starter, butter, rye flour, whole wheat flour, and all purpose flour, and stir until dough pulls away from side of bowl. Add in salt.

Flour work area and knead dough for 5-8 minutes.

Cover and let rise until doubled.

Punch dough down. Form into desired shape (loaf or rolls).

Combine **Oatmeal** flakes, **molasses**, and **caraway** seeds. Top loaf or rolls with **Oatmeal** mixture, and let rise 30-60 minutes.

Heat oven to 375 degrees.

Bake loaves 30-40 minutes; rolls 12-15 minutes.

Salads

Caraway Coleslaw

(8 servings; Polish ancestors' recipe)

Coleslaw

3 cups cabbage, shredded

1 large (or 2 small) **carrots**, grated

1 green bell pepper, finely chopped

Coleslaw dressing (recipe below)

Mix together cabbage, **carrot(s)**, and green pepper.

Toss with dressing.

Coleslaw Dressing

½ cup mayonnaise

½ tsp dry mustard

1 tbsp sugar

2 tbsp lemon juice

1 small onion, grated

1 tsp **Caraway** seeds

1 tbsp vinegar

Salt, to taste

Ground black pepper, to taste

Mix together all ingredients. Refrigerate until ready to use.

Sauerkraut Salad

(4 servings; Polish ancestors' recipe)

1¼ cups sugar
½ tsp celery seeds
½ cup salad oil
1 tbsp **Caraway** seeds
1 tbsp prepared mustard
½ cup vinegar
4 cups sauerkraut, rinsed and drained
¼ cup celery, diced
1 cup onion, diced
¼ cup green bell pepper, diced

To make dressing, mix sugar, celery seeds, oil, **Caraway** seeds, mustard, and vinegar in a small saucepan. Bring to a boil and cook until sugar melts. Chill dressing several hours or overnight.

In a salad bowl, mix sauerkraut, celery, onion, and green pepper.

Add dressing and toss to coat.

Serve.

Soups

Roux Soup

(4 servings)

¼ tsp **Caraway** seeds
1 tbsp sunflower oil
2 tbsp flour
1 tsp sweet paprika
3 cups water (divided)
Salt, to taste
1 tsp wine vinegar
Croutons, as desired

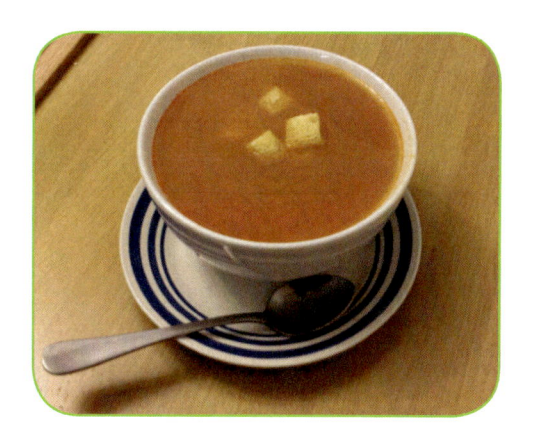

In a soup pan, sauté **Caraway** seeds in hot oil until seeds begin to "crackle."

Add flour. Whisk constantly while bubbling over medium heat until flour is no longer lumpy. Stir in paprika.

Add 1 cup water and allow to come to a boil without stirring. When boiling, stir until mixture blends smoothly.

Slowly add remaining water, beating well after each addition. Cook for additional 5 minutes.

Add vinegar and season with salt and pepper.

Serve with croutons.

Entrees

Beef Cabbage Rolls

(8 servings; Polish ancestors' recipe)

1 (28-ounce) can diced tomatoes

1 sprig oregano, leaves only, roughly chopped

2 tbsp sweet pickle relish

2 tsp sriracha (Thai hot sauce) (divided)

½ tsp allspice

1 tbsp cider vinegar

16-20 outer layer cabbage leaves, blanched

1 tbsp hot and spicy **Garlic** oil

½ medium onion, chopped

½ green pepper, chopped

3 **Garlic** cloves, pressed or finely minced

¼ pound baby bok choy, cut into long thin strips

2 tsp sugar

2 tsp ground mustard

1 tsp **Caraway** seeds

½ tsp celery seeds

1 pound cooked ground beef, drained

2 cups cooked **rice**

Salt to taste

Fresh cracked black pepper to taste

4 ounces mild cheddar cheese, grated

Olive oil, for drizzling

Preheat oven to 350 degrees.

Pour tomatoes into a medium bowl. Lightly crush by hand. Add oregano, sweet pickle relish, 1 tsp sriracha, and allspice. Mix and set sauce aside.

Using medium heat, bring a large pot of salted water to a boil. Add vinegar. Blanche cabbage leaves, several at a time and drain on paper towels. With a paring knife, cut main stalk vein out of each cabbage leaf in a triangle fashion.

Heat a cast iron skillet or sauté pan over medium-high heat and add **Garlic** oil. Add onions, peppers, **Garlic**, bok choy, sugar, mustard, 1 tsp sriracha, **Caraway** seeds, and celery seeds. Sauté until vegetables are softened and aromatic, approximately 4 minutes.

Add ground beef and stir to blend well. Fold in **rice** and remove from heat. Season with salt and pepper.

In a medium sized glass baking dish, ladle enough sauce on bottom just to coat.

On each blanched cabbage leaf, place 1 tsp cheddar cheese in middle of leaf and scoop ¼ cup (loosely packed) **rice** mixture on top. Fold sides, then roll. Place cabbage roll in baking dish, seam side down. Repeat until all cabbage leaves have been rolled and placed in baking dish.

Pour remaining sauce over cabbage rolls and cover tightly with foil. (If making ahead, this is a good place to stop.)

Bake for 1½ hours or until cabbage leaf is easily pierced with a fork. Remove foil and bake an additional 10-15 minutes for slight browning.

Remove from oven and allow to rest 10 minutes before serving.

Drizzle with olive oil and garnish with cheese, if desired.

Polish Way

Instead of tomato sauce, use a refrigerated package or large can of sauerkraut.

Depending upon desired sourness of the golobki (Polish name for cabbage rolls), sauerkraut juice may be drained. Add enough water and/or juice to cover the golobki.

Beer Beef Stew

(6-8 servings)

¼ cup flour

2 pounds boneless chuck roast, trimmed and cut into 1-inch cubes

1 tsp salt (divided)

2 tbsp canola oil (divided)

1 tbsp butter (divided)

1 large onion, chopped

1 tbsp tomato paste

4 cups beef broth

1 (12-ounce) can **Beer**

1 tbsp raisins

1 tsp **Caraway** seeds

½ tsp ground black pepper

1½ cups **carrots**, diagonally sliced ½-inch thick

1½ cups parsnips, diagonally sliced ½-inch thick

1 cup turnips, peeled and cubed ½-inch thick

Place flour and ½ tsp salt in a shallow dish. Dredge beef in flour mixture.

In a large pot, heat 1 tbsp oil and 1½ tsp butter.

Brown half of beef. Remove beef from pot. Add remaining 1 tbsp oil and 1½ tsp butter, and brown other half of beef. Remove from pot.

Add onion to pot; cook until tender, stirring occasionally.

Stir in tomato paste; cook 1 minute, stirring frequently.

Stir in broth and **Beer**, scraping pan to loosen browned bits. Return meat to pan.

Stir in ½ tsp salt, raisins, **Caraway** seeds, and pepper; bring to a boil. Cover, reduce heat, and simmer 1 hour, stirring occasionally.

Add **carrots**, parsnips, and turnips. Return to a boil. Cover, reduce heat to low, and simmer until vegetables are tender.

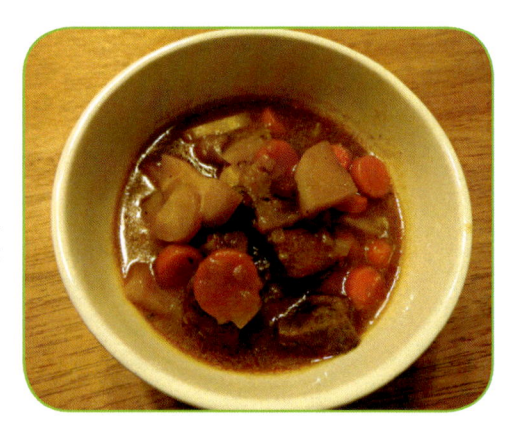

Eggplant and Chickpea Stew

(4 servings)

2 large yellow onions, diced
8 cloves **Garlic**, smashed and chopped
1 (1-inch) **Ginger** root, minced
¼ cup olive oil
1 large eggplant cubed (½-1 inch)
½ tsp **Caraway** seeds
¼ tsp ground **cumin**
½ tsp allspice
½ tsp salt
½ tsp ground black pepper
½ tsp cayenne pepper
1 (14½ ounce) can **chickpeas** (garbanzo beans), drained
1 cup green **peas** (fresh or frozen, thawed)
1 (16 ounce) can tomato sauce
1 (16 ounce) can stewed tomatoes
4 servings brown or white **rice**, cooked

In a soup pot, sauté onions, **Garlic**, and **Ginger** in olive oil until onions are translucent.

Add eggplant and sauté until partly browned.

Add **Caraway** seeds, ground **cumin**, allspice, salt, black pepper, and cayenne pepper, and mix.

Add **chickpeas**, **peas**, tomato sauce, and stewed tomatoes. Bring to a boil; simmer for 30 minutes. Add water if needed.

Serve over **rice**.

Pork Shoulder with Sauerkraut and Apples

(8 servings)

1 (4-5 pound) boneless pork shoulder roast
Salt, to taste

Freshly ground black pepper, to taste

2 tbsp butter, unsalted

2 tbsp canola oil

1 yellow onion, thinly sliced

3 Golden Delicious apples, peeled, halved, and cored

½ cup dry white wine (such as Chardonnay)

2 pounds sauerkraut, squeezed dry

¼ cup dark brown sugar, firmly packed

1 tbsp **Caraway** seeds

1 Golden Delicious apple, peeled, cored, and sliced, as garnish

Trim away any large pockets of fat on the roast. Season generously with salt and pepper. Starting at thinner end of meat, roll up pork. Tie securely with kitchen twine.

In a skillet over medium-high heat, melt butter with canola oil. Add roast and brown on all sides, turning frequently. Transfer pork to a platter.

Add onion and halved apples to skillet and sauté until lightly browned. Transfer apple mixture to a bowl.

Pour off fat from skillet. Return skillet to medium-high heat, add wine, and deglaze pan, stirring with a wooden spoon to scrape up the browned bits from pan bottom.

See below for different methods to cook roast.

Oven Method

Preheat oven to 325 degrees.

Cover bottom of a large Dutch oven with sauerkraut.

Sprinkle with brown sugar and **Caraway** seeds.

Place pork on top and surround with apple mixture. Pour in wine mixture.

Cover and bake until pork is fork-tender and shreds easily, approximately 4-5 hours.

Slow-Cooker Method

Cover bottom of a slow cooker with sauerkraut.

Sprinkle with brown sugar and **Caraway** seeds.

Place pork on top and surround with apple mixture. Pour in wine mixture.

Cover and cook on low until pork is fork-tender and shreds easily, approximately 8-10 hours.

After pork is done:

Transfer pork to a carving board.

Using a sharp knife, cut pork crosswise into slices approximately 1/2-inch thick, removing twine as you slice.

Place sauerkraut on a large platter and top with pork slices.

Surround with raw, sliced apples and serve immediately.

Sausage and Apple Rolls

(12 rolls)

2 tsp olive oil

1 small red onion, finely chopped

1 **Garlic** clove, crushed

10 ounces pork sausage

6 ounces ground pork

1 tsp **Caraway** seeds

2 Granny Smith apples, grated

2 sheets fresh or frozen puff pastry, partially thawed

1 egg, slightly beaten

Garlic butter (recipe below)

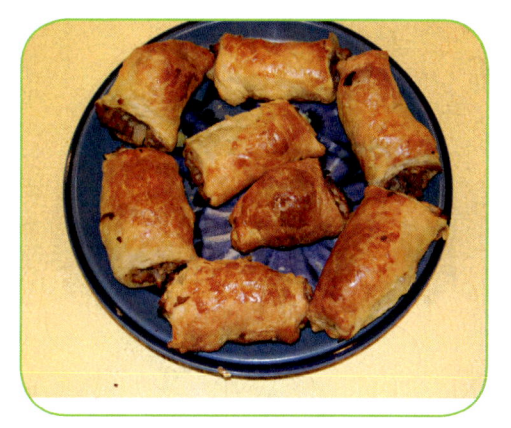

Preheat oven to 400 degrees.

Heat oil in skillet over medium heat. Add onion and **Garlic**. Cook, stirring for 2 minutes or until tender. Set aside to cool.

Remove sausage from casing. Add ground pork, **Caraway** seeds, and onion mixture.

Remove excess moisture from grated apples. Add apples to meat mixture. Season with salt and pepper. Mix well.

Place puff pastry sheets on counter and cut in thirds horizontally (makes six total pieces).

Spoon ⅙ of the sausage/apple mixture along one long edge of each pastry piece.

Brush pastry edges with beaten egg and roll up tightly to enclose filling.

Cut each roll in half. Brush tops with egg.

Place rolls, seam side down, on a baking tray lined with baking paper.

Bake sausage rolls for 40 minutes or until golden and puffed.

Serve with cooked vegetables topped with **garlic** butter (recipe below).

Note: To freeze rolls, allow to cool completely. Place in a single layer in snap-lock freezer bags. Seal and freeze for up to 6 months. To reheat, place frozen rolls on a baking tray. Heat in 350 degree oven for 20 minutes or until heated through.

Garlic Butter

½ cup butter, softened

½ tbsp **Garlic**, minced

⅛ cup grated Parmesan cheese

½ tbsp **Garlic** powder

½ tsp Italian seasoning

¼ tsp ground black pepper

¼ tsp ground paprika

In a small bowl, combine butter, **garlic**, and Parmesan cheese.

Season with **Garlic** powder, Italian seasoning, pepper, and paprika. Mix until smooth.

Refrigerate.

Sides

Cheesy Fried Rice

(4 servings)

2 tsp vegetable oil

1 onion, chopped

3 green chilies, slit lengthwise

½ tsp **Ginger Garlic** paste (recipe below)

2 curry leaves

4 cloves

1 small cinnamon stick

½ tsp ground cardamon

½ tsp **Caraway** seeds

1 pinch **turmeric** powder

½ cup large curd cottage cheese, compressed and drained

¼ tsp garam masala powder (recipe below)

2 cups **rice** (cooked so grains are hard and can be separated)

Salt, to taste

2 tbsp **Coriander seeds**

Heat oil in pan. Add chopped onion and green chilies, and sauté until soft.

Add **Ginger Garlic** paste, curry leaves, cloves, cinnamon stick, cardamom, **Caraway** seeds, and **turmeric** powder, and sauté for 2 additional minutes.

Add cottage cheese and garam masala powder, and sauté for 1 minute.

Add **rice** and salt. Sauté for 2-3 minutes.

To serve, garnish with **Coriander seeds**.

Ginger Garlic Paste

½ cup **Ginger**, peeled and sliced

⅜ cup **Garlic**, peeled and sliced

⅛ tsp **turmeric** powder

⅜ tsp salt

½ tbsp water

½ tbsp vinegar

½ tbsp olive oil, warmed

Blend all ingredients into a smooth paste.

Store in tightly closed bottle in refrigerator up to six months.

Garam Masala (or store bought)

1 tbsp ground **cumin**

1½ tsp ground **Coriander**

1½ tsp ground cardamom

1½ tsp ground black pepper

1 tsp ground cinnamon

½ tsp ground cloves

½ tsp ground nutmeg

Mix all ingredients together.

Place mix in an airtight container and store in a cool, dry place.

German Style Red Cabbage

(8 servings; Nice family recipe)

1 cup onions, chopped

2 tbsp butter

1 medium head red cabbage

¼ cup sugar (or more, to taste)

5 tbsp cider vinegar

Salt, to taste

Ground black pepper, to taste

4-5 bay leaves

1 serving ground cloves, to taste

½ tsp **Caraway** seeds

3 apples, peeled and chopped

1 tbsp strawberry jam (optional)

Sauté chopped onion in butter.

Add cabbage, sugar, cider vinegar, salt, pepper, bay leaves, cloves, and **Caraway** seeds. Mix together.

Add apples. For additional sweetness, add 1 heaping tbsp of strawberry jam.

Simmer for 30 minutes.

Serve.

Desserts

Caraway Cake

(1 cake)

1½ cups flour
1 tsp baking powder
1 small **carrot**, grated
3 tbsp **Caraway** seeds
5 ounces butter, unsalted, softened
¾ cup sugar
3 eggs, beaten
4 tbsp orange marmalade
Zest of 1 orange
Juice from 1 orange

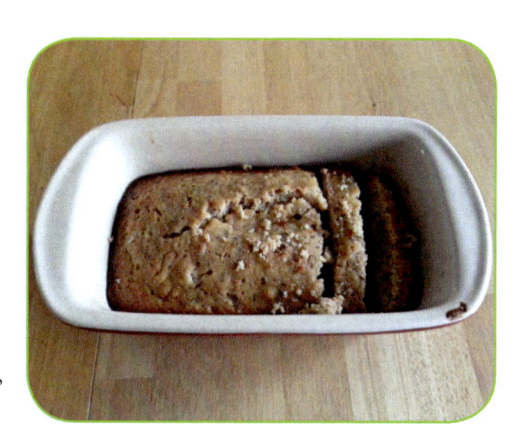

Preheat oven to 350 degrees.

Mix together flour, baking powder, **carrot**, and **Caraway** seeds.

In a separate bowl, cream butter and sugar, gradually adding in eggs.

Add egg mixture to flour mixture.

Fold in marmalade, zest, and juice.

Pour mixture into buttered loaf pan and bake for 45 minutes.

Chasteberry

Unfortunately, I could only find two **Chasteberry** recipes. The dried fruit extract could be added to other recipes as desired. Since the berries have a pepper-like taste and smell, one might try substituting **Chasteberry** for regular pepper in recipes. This is the best I can come up with as a pharmacist.

Chaste Tree Fruit, Chasteberry, Vitex (Agni casti fructus)

Type: Major galactogogue

Medicinal Dose: 30 mg to 40 mg daily as an alcoholic extract (50%-70% alcohol)

Other Uses: To treat breast pain dysmenorrhea

Caution: Herb may cause rash; extract form has high alcohol content, although amount consumed is very small.

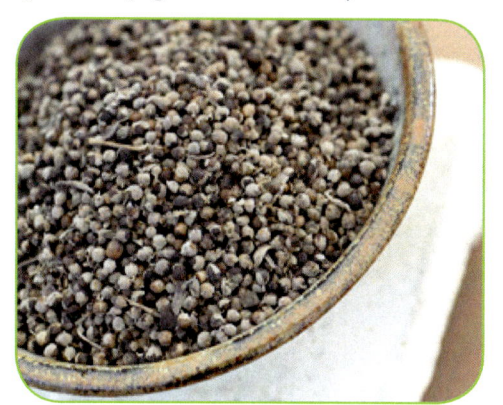

Beverages

Chasteberry Tea

(1 serving)

1 tsp **Chasteberry** berries
8 ounces boiling water
1 tsp honey

Warm a teapot.
Add **Chasteberry** berries. Pour boiling water over berries.
Let steep for 5-10 minutes.
Strain into a cup.
Sweeten with honey.

Salads

Fruit Salad with Chasteberry Dressing

(8 servings)

2 bunches fresh mint, washed
1 cup water, plus 4 tbsp
½ cup caster sugar (finely ground granulated sugar)
½ cup balsamic vinegar
½ tsp black peppercorns
1½ tsp **Chasteberry** seeds (divided)
4 tsp cornstarch
6 large peaches, blanched, peeled, pitted, and sliced
1 honeydew melon, peeled, deseeded, and cubed
1 small pineapple, peeled, cored, and cubed
1 lb strawberries, hulled and halved, if large
1 lb **Red Raspberries**

Strip the leaves from one bunch of the mint. Place leaves in pan with 1 cup water, sugar, balsamic vinegar, peppercorns, and 1 tsp **Chasteberry** seeds. Bring mixture to a boil, reduce to simmer, and cook for 5 minutes.

Place cornstarch in a small bowl and mix with 4 tbsp water to form a smooth slurry.

Add cornstarch mixture to balsamic vinegar mixture in saucepan. Whisk until smooth. Bring to a boil, take off the heat, and set aside to cool for 10 minutes. Pass through fine-meshed sieve and set dressing aside.

Combine peaches, melon, pineapple, and strawberries in a bowl.

Pour dressing over fruit and toss to combine.

Shred other bunch of mint leaves.

Add **Red Raspberries** and shredded mint leaves to fruit mixture, and toss gently to mix.

Garnish with ½ tsp coarsely-ground **Chasteberry** seeds and serve.

Coriander

Coriander is the seed of cilantro. Avoid **Coriander** if you are allergic to celery (so far I have only met one person allergic to celery).

Coriander, Cilantro (Coriandri fructus)

Type: Minor galactogogue

Medicinal Dose: 3 grams daily as tea

Other Uses: Antiflatulent, diuretic, and mild antidiabetic

Caution: Herb may rarely cause photosensitivity; avoid herb if allergic to celery; avoid large amounts of herb.

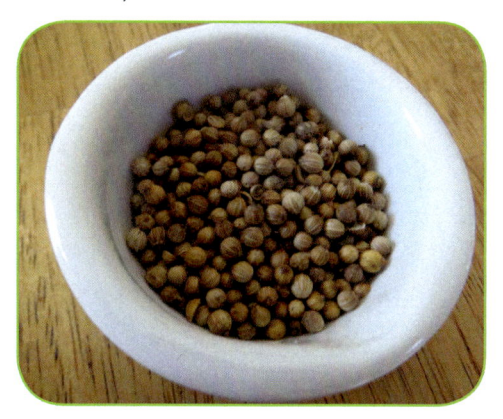

Appetizers

Deviled Egg Dip

(12 servings)

12 hardboiled large eggs

3½ ounces vegetable oil

2 tbsp fresh **Coriander** (cilantro) leaves, minced

5 ounces sour cream

Prepared mustard, to taste

Salt, to taste

Lemon juice, to taste

Slice hardboiled eggs in half. Remove eggs yolks.

Mash yolks with a fork.

Add oil to mashed yolks, a small amount at a time, and beat to create a smooth mixture.

Stir in minced **Coriander** (cilantro) leaves, sour cream, mustard, salt, and lemon juice.

Spoon yolk dip into holes on sliced egg whites.

Refrigerate until ready to serve.

Salads

Avocado Grapefruit Salad with Coriander Dressing

(2 servings)

2 pink grapefruits

3 tbsp grapefruit juice

2 tbsp olive oil

1 tbsp shallot, minced

1 tsp soy sauce

½ tsp honey

¼ tsp sesame oil

1 tsp grated fresh **Ginger** peel

1 tsp **Coriander seeds**

Salt and pepper, to taste

2 cups (packed) mixed baby greens

1 small avocado, halved, pitted, and peeled

Cut off peel and white pith from 1 grapefruit. Cut grapefruit crosswise into 4 slices.

Juice second grapefruit. Whisk 3 tbsp grapefruit juice, olive oil, shallot, soy sauce, honey, sesame oil, **Ginger**, and **Coriander seeds** in small bowl to make dressing. Season with salt and pepper.

Toss greens with 2 tbsp dressing in medium bowl and divide between two plates.

Arrange two grapefruit slices and half an avocado on top of the greens on each plate. Spoon remaining dressing over grapefruit and avocado.

Cabbage Salad

(4 servings)

1 tsp salt

1 tsp brown (or white) sugar

6 tsp fresh lemon juice

2 tbsp vegetable oil

½ tsp mustard seeds

½ tsp **cumin** seeds

4 tbsp **Coriander seeds**

¼ teaspoon **turmeric** powder

1 tbsp hot green chili, seeded and minced

1 medium cabbage (inner leaves only), finely shredded (approximately 6 cups)

4 medium tomatoes, finely chopped

½ cup ground, roasted peanuts

⅔ cup grated fresh **coconut**

In a small bowl, whisk salt, sugar, and lemon juice.

Sauté mustard seeds in oil in a small pan over moderate heat until they crackle.

Add **cumin** seeds, **Coriander seeds**, **turmeric**, and green chili. Sauté until the **cumin** seeds turn a darker shade. Remove from heat and let cool.

Add spices to lemon juice dressing and mix well.

In a large bowl, combine cabbage, tomatoes, ground peanuts, and **coconut**. Add dressing and gently toss to coat well.

Chill at least 1 hour (the longer, the better) in refrigerator to bring out taste.

Soups

Brown Lentil Soup

(8 servings)

2 tbsp olive oil

1 cup onion, finely chopped

½ cup **carrot**, finely chopped

½ cup celery, finely chopped

1 pound **lentils**, rinsed

2 large russet potatoes, cut into ½-inch cubes

1 cup tomatoes, peeled and chopped

2 quarts **chicken broth**

½ tsp freshly ground **Coriander**

½ tsp freshly ground toasted **cumin**

2 tsp salt

Ground black pepper, to taste

1 (10-ounce) package frozen **spinach**

2 scallions, finely chopped

In a large pot, heat olive oil over medium heat. Add onion, **carrot**, and celery. Cook until onions are translucent, approximately 6-7 minutes.

Add **lentils**, potatoes, tomatoes, broth, **Coriander**, **cumin**, salt, and pepper.

Bring to a boil. Reduce heat to low, cover, and simmer approximately 25 minutes.

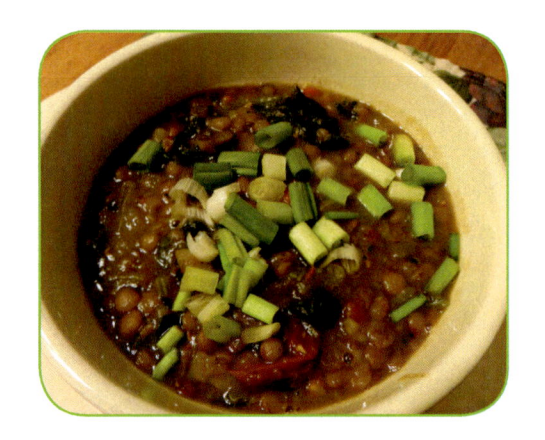

Add **spinach**, stirring occasionally until **spinach** thaws and mixes with soup. Simmer until **lentils** are tender, approximately 10-15 minutes.

To serve, top with chopped scallions.

Carrot Sweet Potato Soup

(8 servings)

2 tbsp olive oil

½ cup shallot, finely chopped

2 **Garlic** cloves, finely chopped

2 tsp **Coriander seeds**, crushed

1 tsp ground **turmeric**

¼ tsp ground cayenne

1 tsp orange zest (colored portion of peel)

1½ pounds **carrots**, cleaned and thinly sliced

1 cup dry white wine

2 cups **chicken stock**

1½ cups (1 large) **sweet potato**, peeled and cubed

3 tbsp orange juice (from orange previously used for zest)

¼ tsp salt

¼ tsp ground black pepper

2 tbsp fresh cilantro (**Coriander**), minced

1 tbsp heavy cream or sour cream or yogurt

In heavy pot, heat oil. Sauté shallot until translucent.

Add **Garlic** and sauté until tender, but not brown.

Add **Coriander**, **turmeric**, cayenne, and orange zest. Stir well to coat onions and **garlic**. Sauté until fragrant.

Add **carrots** and sauté for 3-4 minutes, stirring frequently.

Add wine and deglaze pan. Allow mixture to boil for 3 minutes.

Add **chicken stock**, sweet potato, orange juice, salt, and pepper. Reduce heat to simmer. Cover and let simmer until **carrots** and **sweet potatoes** are tender.

Use an immersion blender to liquefy the soup.

Add chopped cilantro leaves. Stir well. Taste and adjust seasonings.

To serve, garnish with a drizzle of heavy cream, sour cream, or plain yogurt.

Entrees

BBQ Pork Spareribs

(6 servings)

3 tbsp coarse salt

3 tbsp freshly ground black pepper

¼ cup brown sugar

2 tbsp each of paprika, chili powder, **cumin**, ground **Coriander**, cayenne pepper

1 tbsp **Ginger**

2 racks pork spareribs, approximately 3 pounds each

1 cup ketchup

⅓ cup cider vinegar

¼ cup brown sugar

¼ cup orange juice

2 tbsp brown mustard

½ tsp Liquid Smoke

Salt, to taste

Ground black pepper, to taste

Preheat oven to 200 degrees.

In a small bowl, combine salt, pepper, brown sugar, paprika, chili powder, **cumin**, **Coriander**, cayenne pepper, and **Ginger**. Coat ribs with this mixture.

Place ribs on in a single layer on baking sheets. Roast until meat is tender, approximately 3 hours.

When ribs are almost finished in oven, preheat grill to low with grate set high.

Remove ribs from oven and place on grill. Grill for 10-20 minutes, being careful not to burn ribs.

In a small bowl, combine ketchup, vinegar, brown sugar, orange juice, mustard, and Liquid Smoke to make a sauce.

Brush ribs with sauce during final minute of cooking.

Coriander Lemon Chicken

(8 servings)

    3-4 lemons, juiced

    3-4 **Garlic** cloves

    2 tsp dried oregano

    2 tsp paprika powder

    2 tsp **cumin** powder

    2 tsp **Coriander** powder

    1 tbsp extra-virgin olive oil

    1 chili pepper, to taste

    1 tsp ground black pepper

    1 tsp salt

    1 medium-sized cooked chicken, boiled or roasted, and shredded

    ⅓-½ cup **Coriander seeds**

Place lemon juice, **Garlic**, oregano, paprika, **cumin**, **Coriander** powder, olive oil, chili pepper, black pepper, and salt in a bowl and mix.

Add shredded chicken. Toss to coat with dressing.

Add **Coriander seeds**. Mix.

Let chicken marinate in refrigerator for 60 minutes or longer.

Serve in tacos, on sandwiches, or as a salad.

Note: Recipe makes approximately 3 ounces marinade (if more marinade is desired, add another lemon and an extra pinch (approximately ¼ teaspoon) of spices.

Creole Chicken Livers

(4 servings)

    3 tbsp wine vinegar

    5 tbsp olive oil (divided)

    1 tbsp lemon juice

    2 **Garlic** cloves, crushed

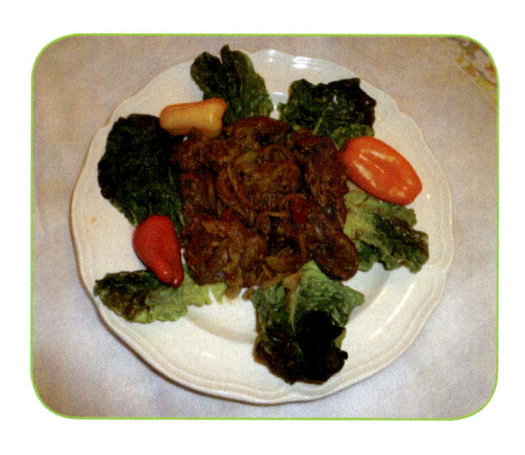

2 red chilies, seeded and chopped

1 tsp ground **cumin**

1 tsp ground **Coriander**

Salt, to taste

Freshly ground black pepper, to taste

1 pound chicken livers, trimmed

1 tbsp butter or margarine

1 onion, thinly sliced

1 tbsp tomato paste

1 tbsp Worcestershire sauce

½ cup **chicken stock**

2 tbsp brandy or Haitian rum

Ground **Coriander** as garnish

Combine wine vinegar, 3 tbsp olive oil, lemon juice, **Garlic**, chilies, **cumin**, **Coriander**, and salt and pepper. Marinate chicken livers in this mixture for 2 hours. Drain livers and set aside, reserving the marinade.

Heat 2 tbsp olive oil and butter. Add onion and sauté until soft.

Add chicken livers. Cook over high heat for 2 minutes.

Reduce heat and add tomato paste, Worcestershire sauce, **chicken stock**, reserved marinade, and brandy or rum. Simmer gently for 5 minutes.

Before serving, sprinkle with ground **Coriander**.

Serve with crusty bread, baked potato, baked sweet potato, **rice**, and/or red, orange, and/or yellow sweet peppers.

Fish Tacos with Lime-Cilantro Salsa

(4 servings)

1 tsp ground **cumin**

1 tsp ground **Coriander**

½ tsp paprika

¼ tsp ground red pepper

⅛ tsp salt

⅛ tsp **Garlic** powder

1½ pounds swai (similar to catfish), tilapia, or red snapper fillets

Cooking spray, as needed

8 (6-inch) corn tortillas

¼ cup green onions, thinly sliced

1 tbsp **Coriander seeds**

3 tbsp fat-free mayonnaise

3 tbsp reduced-fat sour cream

1 tsp lime zest

1½ tsp fresh lime juice

¼ tsp salt

1 **Garlic** clove, minced

¼ cup **lettuce**, shredded

Preheat oven to 425 degrees.

Combine **cumin**, **Coriander**, paprika, red pepper, salt and **Garlic** powder in a bowl; sprinkle spice mixture evenly over both sides of fish.

Place fish on a baking sheet coated with cooking spray. Bake in oven for 9 minutes or until fish flakes easily when a fork is inserted. When fish is done, break into pieces with a fork.

Heat tortillas according to package directions.

Combine green onions, **Coriander seeds**, mayonnaise, sour cream, lime zest, lime juice, salt, and **garlic** in a small bowl to make salsa.

Divide fish evenly among tortillas.

Top with **lettuce** and salsa.

Marinated Prime Rib Roast

(12 servings)

¼ cup soy sauce

⅔ cup Worcestershire sauce

8 **Garlic** cloves, minced

1 tbsp Liquid Smoke

¼ cup olive oil

1½ cups beef broth

1 (10-ounce) can pineapple tidbits, with juice

1 tbsp mustard powder

1 tsp ground cloves

1 tsp **Coriander** powder

1 tsp onion powder

2 bay leaves

1 tsp ground black pepper

½ cup brown sugar

1 (8-pound) prime rib roast

¾ tsp coarse salt

¼ cup flour

In a large bowl, mix together soy sauce, Worcestershire sauce, minced **garlic**, Liquid Smoke, olive oil, beef broth, pineapple tidbits with juice, mustard powder, ground cloves, **Coriander** powder, onion powder, bay leaves, black pepper, and brown sugar to make marinade.

Prick holes all over roast. Rub roast with salt and flour.

Place roast in a roasting pan. Pour marinade over roast. Cover and refrigerate for at least 3 hours, basting at least twice.

Preheat oven to 400 degrees.

Cook roast for 1 hour. Remove aluminum foil, baste, and reduce heat to 325 degrees. Cook for another hour. Use a meat thermometer to test for doneness. For medium rare, the thermometer should read at least 140 degrees, for well done - 170 degrees.

Remove roasting pan from oven. Let roast rest for approximately 30 minutes before slicing.

Use drippings for sauce.

Moroccan Stuffed Potatoes

(6 servings)

6 medium potatoes of uniform size, scrubbed

1 pound ground beef

½ tsp salt

½ tsp ground black pepper

⅔ tsp Baharat spice (recipe below)

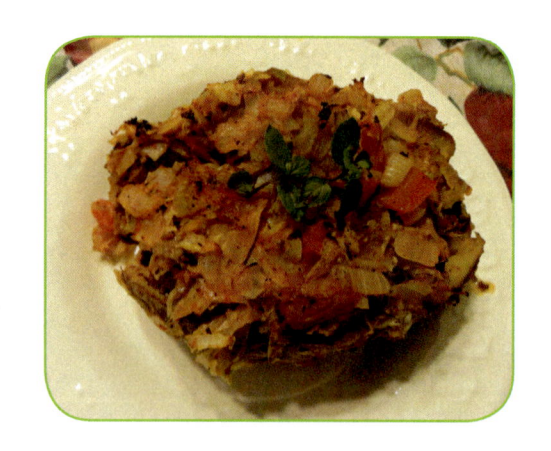

⅓ tsp ground **turmeric**

½ tbsp sweet paprika

½ tsp ground cinnamon

1 chili pepper, to taste

½ tsp ground **Ginger**

4 stalks celery, coarsely chopped

Vegetable oil

1 large onion, chopped

4 **Garlic** cloves, crushed

3 tbsp tomato paste

½ cup tomatoes, diced

¼ cabbage, cut into coarse chunks

4 cups **chicken stock**

1 tsp salt or to taste

¼ tsp pepper or to taste

3 tbsp celery leaves, chopped

Preheat oven to 425 degrees. Using a fork, poke several holes in potatoes to release steam while cooking. Lay potatoes on rack in oven and cook for 60 minutes or until tender.

Combine meat with salt, black pepper, Baharat spice, **turmeric**, paprika, cinnamon, chili pepper, and **Ginger**. Mix well. Cover. Place in the refrigerator for 30 minutes to allow meat to absorb spices.

After 30 minutes, brown ground meat until crumbly. Set aside.

In a large pot, sauté celery in oil until tender. Add onion and **Garlic**, and cook until onion is translucent. Add tomato paste, chopped tomato, cabbage, and **chicken stock**. Season lightly with salt and pepper. Cook sauce until cabbage is tender.

When baked potatoes are tender, remove from oven and reduce oven temperature to 350 degrees. Let potatoes sit for a few minutes.

Put potatoes in a greased casserole dish. Cut a slit in each potato from one end to the other. Stuff potatoes with ground meat, then cover with cabbage sauce.

Return potatoes to oven and bake for 30 minutes.

Garnish with celery leaves and serve.

Baharat Spice Mix (or you can use store bought)

1 tbsp cardamom

1 tbsp ground black pepper

½ tbsp allspice

1 tbsp cinnamon

1 tbsp dry **Ginger**

½ tbsp nutmeg

2 tsp ground **cumin**

2 tsp ground **Coriander**

Mix ground and powdered spices.
Stir well and keep in a tight-lidded jar.

Slow Roast Pork

(10-12 servings)

2 tbsp **Coriander seeds**

2 tbsp **Fennel** seeds

3 **Garlic** cloves, chopped

1 tbsp salt

1 tbsp pepper

Extra-virgin olive oil, as needed to make paste

1 (5-6 pound) pork shoulder

3 apples, quartered

3 branches **Fennel** tops

1 cup onions, chopped

3 cups dry white wine

Preheat oven to 250 degrees.

Using a mortar and pestle, crush **Coriander seeds** and **Fennel** seeds. Add **Garlic** cloves, salt, and pepper, and mash together. Add enough olive oil to form a paste. Rub paste on all sides of pork.

Place apples, **Fennel**, and onion in the bottom of a deep, lidded pan. Pour wine over fruit and vegetables.

Place pork on top and cover pan. Cook in oven for 10 hours or overnight.

Remove pork from pan, place on a cutting board, and cover with aluminum foil to keep warm.

Strain liquid into a saucepan, bring to a boil, and cook until reduced by half.

Slice pork.

Serve covered with reduced sauce.

Sides

Spiced Butternut Squash

(12 servings)

2 tbsp olive oil

1 medium onion, chopped

2 **Garlic** cloves, minced

2 tsp **Coriander**, ground

1 ½ tsp salt

1 tsp **cumin**, ground

¼ tsp red pepper (cayenne), ground

¼ tsp nutmeg, ground

1 tsp cinnamon, ground

2 medium butternut squash (approximately 2 ½ pounds each), peeled and cut into ¾ inch chunks

½ cup water

¼ cup, packed, dark brown sugar

2 tbsp butter or margarine

1 cup fresh cilantro leaves, chopped

In 6-quart saucepan, heat oil over medium heat until hot.

Add onion and cook until tender, approximately 5 minutes.

Add **Garlic** and cook 30 seconds.

Stir in **Coriander**, salt, **cumin**, red pepper, nutmeg, and cinnamon; cook for 1 minute.

Add squash and water. Cook, covered, for 15 minutes or until squash is tender.

Add brown sugar and butter or margarine, and gently stir until squash is well coated.

Serve topped with cilantro leaves.

Dandelion

Dandelions are everywhere. They are one of the most nutritious plants around. Once they start to send up leaves, they will be tasty for about a month. Once the thumb-like bud emerges from the center of the plant, it is too late. The **Dandelion** has gone to seed, and the leaves have become bitter. Wash and clean well before using.

Dandelion (Taraxaci herba)

Type: Minor galactogogue

Medicinal Dose: 5 grams, in capsule form or as tincture or tea, 3 times a day

Other Uses: Antidiabetic and diuretic

Caution: Dandelion may rarely cause contact dermatitis; patients with bile duct blockage, gall bladder problems, or bowel obstruction should not use.

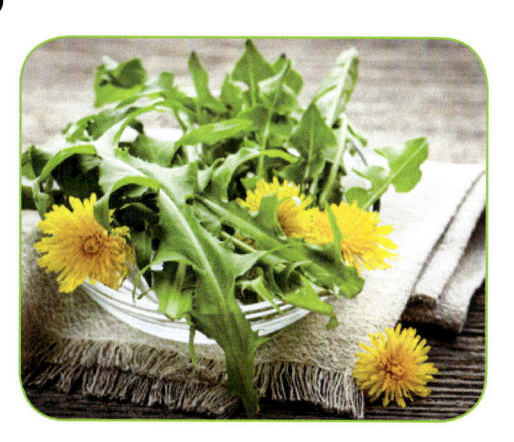

Condiments

Dandelion Honey

(Several jars depending upon size)

250 **Dandelion** flowers

1½ quarts water

1 lemon, finely chopped without seeds

2¼ pounds granulated sugar

Wash **Dandelion** flowers. Place in a pot with water. Add lemon. Cook briefly. Let stand overnight to infuse.

Add sugar to infusion and cook, stirring until mass thickens and sugar melts.

Pour thick honey into jars. Seal properly.

Note: If honey turns to candy, dip jar into cup of warm water, and sugar will dissolve.

Salads

Blue Cheese Dandelion Salad with Citrus Dressing

(4 servings)

4 cups cleaned **Dandelion** greens, chopped

½ cup **Coriander seeds**

½ cup walnuts, chopped

12 grape tomatoes

1 chunk bleu (or blue) cheese, crumbled

½ cup pine nuts

1 lemon, chopped

1 lime, chopped

1 orange, chopped

2 tbsp olive oil

1 tbsp red wine vinegar

1 tbsp cider vinegar

1 peppercorn, ground

1 **Garlic** clove, diced

Toss **Dandelion** greens with **Coriander seeds**, walnuts, grape tomatoes, bleu cheese, and pine nuts in a large bowl.

In a separate bowl, mix lemon, lime, orange, olive oil, red wine vinegar, cider vinegar, peppercorn, and **Garlic** to make dressing.

Just before serving, toss salad with salad dressing.

Dandelion Greens with Pennsylvania Dutch Hot Bacon Dressing

(4 servings)

3 slices bacon

4 cups cleaned **Dandelion** greens, chopped

1 onion, chopped

1 egg, well beaten

1½ tbsp flour

1 cup milk

¼ cup vinegar

¼ cup sugar

½ tsp salt

Cook bacon in skillet until crisp; remove, drain, and chop. Reserve bacon fat in skillet.

Put chopped bacon, **Dandelion** greens, and onion in a large bowl.

Beat egg in small bowl. Add flour, milk, vinegar, sugar, and salt.

Heat skillet with reserved bacon fat. Add egg mixture. Whisk until thickened to make dressing.

Dress **Dandelion** greens with dressing. Serve.

Soups

Hearty Vegetable Soup

(8 servings)

2 tbsp extra-virgin olive oil

1 large onion, minced

4 large **Garlic** cloves, chopped

3 stalks celery, minced

1½ quarts **chicken stock**

1 (28-ounce can) crushed tomatoes with juice

3 medium **carrots**, minced

2 medium potatoes, diced

1-2 tbsp mixed dried herbs (**basil**, marjoram, etc.)

1 can beans (including **green beans**) of choice, liquid removed, rinsed

6 cups cleaned **Dandelion** greens, chopped

Salt, to taste

Freshly ground black pepper, to taste

In a large soup pot, heat oil. Add onions, **Garlic**, and celery, and cook over medium heat until onions are soft.

Add **chicken stock** and tomatoes; simmer for 15 minutes.

Add **carrots**, potatoes, herbs, and beans. Cook until **carrots** and potatoes are just tender, approximately 15 minutes.

Add **Dandelion** greens, and cook until **Dandelion** greens are tender.

Season with salt and pepper.

Spring Vegetable Soup

(8 servings)

2 tbsp extra-virgin olive oil

2 small leeks, trimmed and diced

½ pound **asparagus**, cut in 1-inch pieces

1 cup **peas**, freshly shelled

2 ounces fresh **Dandelion** leaves and/or fresh **Stinging Nettles** leaves

1 tsp salt, plus to taste

8 cups water (divided)

1 pound fresh **spinach**

1 ounce watercress, stems removed

12 ice cubes

Freshly ground black pepper, to taste

8 tbsp ricotta cheese

Extra-virgin olive oil, for drizzling

Heat 2 tbsp extra virgin olive oil in a heavy, 6-quart saucepan.

Sauté leeks, **asparagus**, **peas**, and **Dandelion** and/or **Stinging Nettles** leaves.

Add water and salt. Bring to a boil; reduce heat and simmer until vegetables are tender.

Add **spinach** and watercress, stirring until leaves are wilted, approximately 2 minutes.

Puree using an immersion blender.

Season with salt and pepper to taste.

Garnish each serving with 1 tbsp ricotta cheese and a drizzle of extra-virgin olive oil.

Entrees

Creamy Dandelion Greens and Ham

(4 servings)

1 tsp butter, unsalted

½ pound smoked ham, cut into 4 slices

1 **Garlic** clove, chopped

10 ounces **Dandelion** greens, cleaned and drained

¼ cup low-fat evaporated milk

¼ tsp room temperature red pepper sauce (or Frank's Red Hot)

Heat butter in skillet over medium-high heat. Cook ham on each side until golden brown. Transfer to a platter and keep warm.

Add **Garlic** and cook 1 minute, stirring, until fragrant.

Add **Dandelion** greens and evaporated milk. Cook 4-5 minutes, stirring occasionally, until most of the liquid is absorbed. Season with red pepper sauce.

Place each ham slice on a plate, top with creamed **Dandelion** greens.

Linguine with Dandelion Greens

(4 servings)

½ cup vegetable stock

½ cup onions, diced

2 tsp **Garlic**, finely chopped

2 tsp red pepper flakes (optional)

1½ cups plum tomatoes peeled and diced (fresh or canned)

½ cup tomato juice

6-8 small potatoes, cooked and cut in 1-inch chunks

4 cups cleaned **Dandelion** greens, chopped

½ cup **green beans**, cooked

Salt, to taste

Ground black pepper, to taste

½ pound pasta (shells, penne, linguine, bow-tie), cooked

Heat vegetable stock in skillet over moderate heat.

Add onions, cover, and cook until tender, approximately 10 minutes.

Add **Garlic** and red pepper flakes (optional), and cook 2 minutes longer.

Add tomatoes, tomato juice, potatoes, **Dandelion** greens, and cooked **green beans**.

Cook until **Dandelion** greens are wilted and potatoes are heated through. Season with salt and pepper.

Pour **Dandelion** sauce over cooked pasta and toss to coat.

Serve.

Marinated Chicken with Spinach and Dandelion Greens

(2 servings)

1 tsp soy sauce

¼ tsp honey

½ tsp sesame oil

1 tsp vegetable oil

1 pinch **turmeric** powder

2 chicken thighs

3½ ounces couscous (Middle Eastern semolina)

8½ ounces water

10 raisins

1 spring onion, dark green part removed, minced

1 tbsp extra-virgin olive oil, plus extra to drizzle as garnish

1 tsp balsamic vinegar, plus extra to drizzle as garnish

Salt, to taste

Ground black pepper, to taste

2 cups cleaned **Dandelion** greens, chopped

2 bunches baby **spinach**, chopped

2 plum tomatoes, washed

Preheat oven to 350 degrees.

Mix soy sauce, honey, sesame oil, and vegetable oil together in a bowl; add **turmeric** powder.

Pat chicken dry and place in soy sauce mixture. Cover and marinate approximately 20 minutes.

Place couscous in a bowl. Bring water to a boil and pour over couscous. Allow to sit for 5 minutes. Add raisins and spring onion.

Mix together 1 tbsp olive oil and 1 tsp balsamic vinegar. Pour over couscous and mix well. Season with salt and pepper. Set aside.

Remove chicken from marinade and place on an oven tray.

Roast chicken in lower part of preheated oven for approximately 30-35 minutes, until cooked through and tender.

Cook **Dandelion** greens and **spinach** in lightly salted water, uncovered, for 8-10 minutes. Drain.

Cut plum tomatoes into thin slices and arrange in a circle on serving plate. Spoon couscous onto center of plate.

Place chicken on top of couscous. Top with greens. Drizzle olive oil and balsamic vinegar over greens.

Pasta with Dandelion Greens and Ricotta

(8 servings)

2¼ pounds **Dandelion** greens, washed

¼ cup extra-virgin olive oil

1 **Garlic** clove, chopped

Salt, to taste

Crushed red pepper flakes, to taste

1 pound bucatini (thick spaghetti with hole in center) or penne or macaroni pasta

¼ pound ricotta cheese

⅓ cup grated Parmesan cheese

Cook **Dandelion** greens in lightly salted water, uncovered, for 8-10 minutes. Drain and coarsely chop. Reserve cooking water.

Heat olive oil over medium heat in a sauté or fry pan. Add **Garlic** and **Dandelion** greens. Sauté for 3-4 minutes. Season with salt and red pepper flakes. Remove from the heat.

Bring water from **Dandelion** greens back to a boil and use to cook pasta as instructed on pasta package. Drain and reserve ¾ cup of the liquid.

Return pasta to cooking pot, add ½ **Dandelion** greens and reserved liquid and toss.

Put pasta/**dandelion** mixture in a serving bowl. Top with remaining **Dandelion** greens and ricotta cheese.

Sprinkle with Parmesan cheese and serve.

Pasta with Dandelion Stems

(4 servings)

2 tbsp extra-virgin olive oil

2 ounces Italian bacon (or bacon), coarsely minced

Dandelion stems from 2 pounds of greens, cut into 1½-inch pieces

2 large **Garlic** cloves, thinly sliced

½ pound linguine, cooked until firm

1 tbsp fresh lemon juice

Large pinch crushed red pepper

Salt, to taste

Freshly grated Parmesan cheese, for accompaniment

In a large skillet, heat olive oil. Add bacon and cook over moderately high heat until crisp. Drain bacon on paper towel.

Add **Dandelion** stems to skillet and cook until crispy tender, approximately 5 minutes.

Add **Garlic** and cook until lightly browned, approximately 2 minutes.

In a large, warmed bowl, toss cooked pasta with **Dandelion** stems, lemon juice, and crushed red pepper. Season with salt.

Serve topped with Parmesan cheese.

Ravioli with Dandelion and Fenugreek

(4 servings)

1 bundle **Dandelion** leaves, chopped

½ bundle **Fenugreek** leaves, chopped

12 ounces ricotta cheese or cottage cheese

1 handful grated Parmesan cheese, plus extra for garnish

1 tbsp ground black pepper

1 tbsp ground nutmeg

4 cups flour

4 large eggs

Blanch **Dandelion** and **Fenugreek** leaves. Drain.

In a large bowl, mix **Dandelion** and **Fenugreek** leaves with ricotta cheese in a bowl. Add Parmesan cheese, pepper, and nutmeg.

In another bowl, mix flour and eggs. Add a small amount water, if required, to make a stiff dough.

Either roll out dough very thinly with a rolling pin or use a pasta machine to make two equal size sheets of dough (each sheet should be about 18x26 inches).

Put heaping teaspoons of **Dandelion/Fenugreek** mix 2 inches apart on one sheet of dough, cover with other sheet of dough. Cut around each lump/blob with a pastry cutter to make ravioli. Each piece of ravioli should be about 1-2 inches across (round or square shaped). You should get about 125 raviolis. Make sure edges are pressed closed.

In a large pot of boiling water, boil ravioli until they float. Drain.

To serve, top ravioli with your favorite pasta sauce. Garnish with Parmesan cheese.

Sides

Batter Fried Dandelion

(4 servings)

1 egg, beaten

1 cup low-fat milk

1 cup flour

½ tsp salt

¼ tsp ground black pepper

2 cups **Dandelion** blossoms, washed and patted dry

Vegetable oil, for frying

Beat egg, milk, flour, salt, and pepper in a small bowl.

Dip blossoms in batter to coat.

Heat oil in deep pan to 275 degrees (hot but not smoking). Fry **Dandelion** blossoms until golden brown.

Drain on paper towels and sprinkle with salt.

Creamed Dandelion Leaves

(4 servings)

1 pound fresh **Dandelion** leaves, washed and finely chopped

1 quart water

2 tbsp butter

½ tsp salt

2 tbsp flour

1 cup low-fat milk

Salt, to taste

Ground black pepper, to taste

Put **Dandelion** leaves in a 3-quart saucepan. Add water and salt, and bring to a boil. Lower heat and simmer for 15 minutes. Remove from heat and drain.

Melt butter in a skillet. Add flour and mix to form a smooth paste. Add milk and stir to make a smooth, thick cream. Season with salt and pepper.

Add **Dandelion** leaves and mix well. Simmer for a minute or two to heat through.

Serve with favorite meat.

Dandy Dandelions

(4 servings)

2 bushels of **Dandelion** greens, washed, hard core removed, and chopped

1 drizzle extra-virgin olive oil

1 lemon, juiced

Salt, to taste

Fill large pot with water and bring to a boil. Add **Dandelion** greens and cook approximately 10 minutes. Drain. Rinse briefly in cool water to stop cooking process.

Place in a serving dish. Drizzle with extra-virgin olive oil, lemon juice, and salt.

Serve.

Pennsylvania Dutch Dandelion Greens

(4 servings)

2 slices bacon

4 tbsp flour

3 tbsp sugar

3 tbsp vinegar

1½ cups milk

4 cups **Dandelion** greens, cleaned and chopped

2 hardboiled eggs

Cook bacon in a large skillet; drain bacon and save for garnish.

Add flour to bacon grease in skillet and mix well. Cook for a minute or two until flour starts to brown.

Combine sugar, vinegar, and milk. Add to flour and bacon grease mixture, and cook until thick.

Pour over **Dandelion** greens.

Garnish with sliced eggs and crumbled bacon.

Dill

When I think of **Dill**, I think of Polish **Dill** pickles, **Dill** sauces, **Dill** breads, and **Dill**…

Dill (Anethi fructus)

Type: Minor galactogogue

Medicinal Dose: 3 grams daily as tincture or tea

Other Uses: Antiflatulent and diuretic

Caution: None.

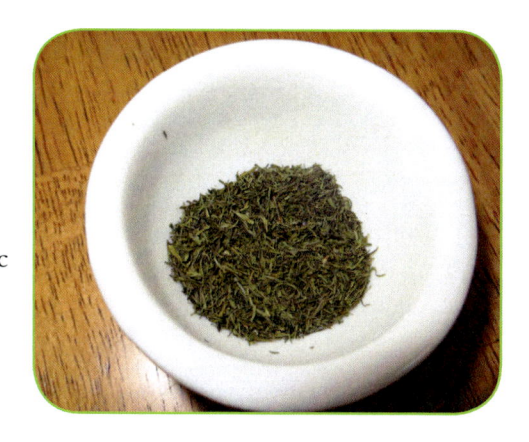

Breads

Dill and Scallion Batter Bread

(1 loaf; Polish ancestors' recipe)

2 tbsp sugar

¼ cup warm water (105-115 degrees)

1¼-ounce package active dry yeast

1 cup plain Greek yogurt

¼ cup fresh **Dill**, chopped

¼ cup scallions, minced

1 large egg

2 tbsp vegetable oil

¼ tsp baking soda

1¼ tsp salt

2½ cups unbleached flour (divided)

In a small bowl, place sugar, warm water, and yeast. Stir to combine. Let sit for approximately 15 minutes to dissolve and bubble.

Grease an 8-inch round casserole dish.

Mix together yogurt, **Dill**, scallions, egg, oil, baking soda, and salt.

Add yeast mixture and 2 cups flour.

Beat well until dough begins to pull away from sides of bowl. Stir in remainder of flour, a small amount at a time, until dough is soft and workable.

Dampen hands, shape dough into a rough ball in mixing bowl.

Transfer dough to prepared dish, flattening it so it covers bottom of dish and is fairly level.

Cover with plastic wrap and let set in a warm, draft-free area. Dough will rise to approximately double its size in approximately 90 minutes.

Preheat oven to 350 degrees.

Bake 25-45 minutes until top is evenly browned. Remove from oven and cool on wire rack.

Yogurt Dill Biscuits

(9 biscuits; Polish ancestors' recipe)

2 cups flour

¼ tsp salt

1 tbsp baking powder

1 tsp baking soda

¼ cup unsalted butter

10 oz plain Greek yogurt

¼ cup fresh **Dill**, roughly chopped, or 1 tsp **Dill**, dried

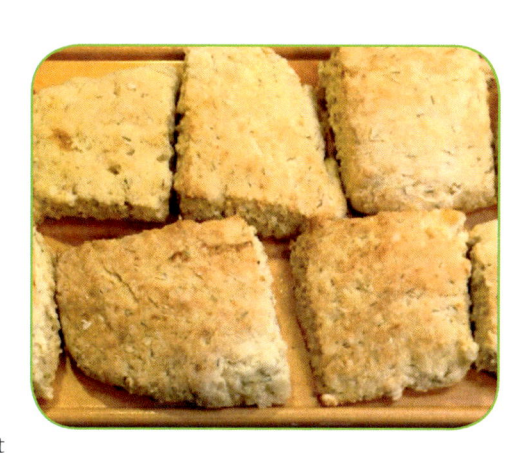

Preheat oven to 450 degrees.

Mix flour, salt, baking powder, and baking soda in a food processor bowl. Add butter and mix, pulsing until very fine meal-like texture results.

Place flour mixture in mixing bowl. Stir in yogurt and **Dill** to form dough.

Place dough on a lightly floured surface and knead 10 times. Press out dough into a square, until it is about ¾-inch thick.

Using a biscuit cutter or small glass, cut dough into biscuits.

Place biscuits on an ungreased baking sheet and bake until golden brown, approximately 7-9 minutes.

Condiments

Dill and Yogurt Salad Dressing

(1 small bowl)

1 cup plain yogurt

2 tbsp fresh **Dill**, finely chopped

2 tbsp honey (or light brown sugar) (optional)

In a small bowl, thoroughly mix yogurt, **Dill**, and honey.

Chill until ready to use.

Polish Dill Pickles

(6 jars)

12 **Garlic** cloves

6 sprigs fresh **Dill** per jar

3 hot peppers with seeds, optional

1 basket pickling cucumbers, washed

3 cups water

1 cup vinegar

3½ tbsp coarse salt

½ hot pepper per jar (optional)

Wash and sterilize 6 medium canning jars.

Place 2 cloves of **Garlic** and 1 sprig of fresh **Dill** at the bottom of each jar. For a spicier pickle, add ½ hot pepper with seeds to each jar.

Pack jars with cucumbers.

Boil water, vinegar, and coarse salt in a saucepan for 5 minutes.

Pour mixture over cucumbers all the way to the top of each jar and seal.

Let cool.

Store in a dark cabinet for a few weeks before opening.

Salads

Arugula with Pears and Dill

(4 servings)

1 bunch arugula, washed and drained

3-4 ripe pears, washed and cut into ¼-inch slices

⅜ cup pear vinegar (check on-line)

1 tbsp walnut oil (check on-line)

1 handful fresh **Dill**, chopped

On four salad plates, place ¼ of arugula on each plate, then arrange ¼ of pear slices on top.

Whisk pear vinegar and walnut oil until it forms an emulsion, and then drizzle over salad.

Garnish with **Dill**.

Cucumber Dill Salad

(2 servings; Polish ancestors' recipe)

1 large cucumber, sliced
¼ cup red onion, sliced
¼ cup sour cream
1 tbsp lemon juice
1 tsp sugar (optional)
1 handful fresh **Dill**, chopped
Salt, to taste
Ground black pepper, to taste

Mix all ingredients together.
Refrigerate for an hour.
Serve.

Dill and Cucumbers in Sour Cream Dressing

(4 servings)

3 long cucumbers, washed
Salt, to taste (divided)
½ pint low-fat sour cream
2 tbsp **rice** vinegar
½ tsp celery seeds
¼ cup scallions, minced
1 tsp sugar
1 handful fresh **Dill**, chopped
Ground black pepper, to taste

Thinly slice cucumbers. Salt lightly. Drain in colander for 30 minutes. Rinse and pat dry.

Combine sour cream, vinegar, celery seeds, scallions, sugar, borage leaves, and salt and pepper (to taste).

Add cucumbers and **Dill** to sour cream mixture and toss lightly.

Refrigerate 1 hour before serving.

Dill and Shallot Potato Salad

(8 servings)

1 small shallot, minced

Salt, to taste

Ground black pepper, to taste

1 scant tsp sugar

3 tbsp cider vinegar

1 tbsp Dijon mustard

⅓ cup canola oil

1 small rib celery, very thinly sliced

1 handful of fresh **Dill**, chopped

Place minced shallot in a bowl. Add salt, pepper, and sugar. Cover with cider vinegar. Add mustard. Whisk in oil. Set aside.

In a large bowl, place cooked potatoes, celery, and **Dill**. Add shallot dressing and toss gently to mix.

Shrimp and Shell Pasta Salad

(4 servings)

8 ounces medium shell, whole grain pasta, cooked per package directions

1 cup frozen petite green **peas**, cooked per package directions, rinsed to cool, and drained

¾ cup celery, diced

⅓ cup onion, finely chopped (or green onions, sliced)

1 (6-ounce) container plain yogurt

⅓ cup mayonnaise

2 tsp Dijon mustard

2 tbsp fresh lemon juice

2 tsp dried **Dill** weed

½ tsp salt

⅛ tsp ground black pepper

2 (4-ounce) cans tiny shrimp, rinsed and drained

4 servings leaf **lettuce**

16 tomato wedges

8 lemon slices

Grated cheese

Place cooked pasta in large bowl with cooked **peas**, celery, and onion.

Mix together yogurt, mayonnaise, mustard, lemon juice, **Dill**, salt, and pepper.

Pour over pasta mixture and mix thoroughly. Lightly fold in shrimp.

Cover and chill for 2 hours.

Serve over leaf **lettuce**, garnished with tomato wedges and lemon slices. Top with grated cheese.

Zucchini Dill Salad

(4 servings)

1 zucchini, green, yellow, or combination, thinly sliced

½ grapefruit

5-6 **Dill** sprigs, washed and stems removed

½ tbsp extra-virgin olive oil

Salt, to taste

1½ tbsp cream

Ground white, black, or chili pepper, to taste

Steam zucchini slices until tender. Put in bowl and refrigerate.

Remove peeling and pith from grapefruit. Cut into wedges, then cut wedges in half.

Mix oil, salt, and cream. Add **Dill** leaves and mix.

In a bowl, gently combine zucchini and grapefruit. Add **Dill** dressing and toss gently.

To serve, top with pepper, to taste.

Soups

Sweet and Sour Cabbage Soup

(8 servings)

9 cups vegetable stock (can use 2 cartons of vegetable stock and add 1 cup water)

1 head cabbage, outer leaves removed, quartered, cored and shredded

1½ cups Spanish onion, diced

½ cup **carrots**, diced

¼ cup celery, diced

1 (28-ounce) can (or two 15-ounce cans) diced tomatoes

8 **Ginger** snaps (regular or gluten free)

2 tsp salt

2 tsp celery salt

½ tsp dried **Dill** weed

¼ cup dark brown sugar

¼ cup cider vinegar

In a large pot, bring stock to a boil.

Add all ingredients, except brown sugar and vinegar. Return to a boil. Reduce heat and simmer until vegetables are tender, approximately 1-1½ hours.

Add brown sugar and vinegar.

Cover and simmer 15 additional minutes.

Entrees

Beef Gyros with Dill Sauce

(6 servings)

½ cup plain Greek yogurt

½ cucumber, peeled, seeded, and chopped finely

¼ tsp salt

1 tbsp fresh lemon juice (from 1/2 lemon)

1 small **Garlic** clove, peeled and minced

1 tbsp fresh **Dill**, chopped

6 (6-inch) pita breads

½ medium onion, chopped

1 tbsp fresh lemon juice (from ½ lemon)

½ tsp salt

¼ tsp freshly ground black pepper

2 tbsp fresh oregano leaves, chopped

3 **Garlic** cloves, peeled and minced

1 pound ground beef

1 tbsp vegetable oil

Shredded **lettuce**

Cucumbers, chopped

Tomatoes, chopped

Onion, chopped

Olives, chopped

Feta cheese

Preheat oven to 350 degrees.

To make **Dill** sauce, combine yogurt, cucumber, salt, lemon juice, **garlic**, and **Dill** in a small bowl. Cover and chill 30 minutes to blend flavors.

Cut off top quarter of each pita, tear into pieces, and set aside. Stack pitas and wrap in foil. Heat pitas in oven for 10-15 minutes.

Combine pita pieces, onion, lemon juice, salt, pepper, oregano, and **Garlic** in a food processor. Process until a smooth paste forms, approximately 30 seconds. Transfer to a large bowl.

Add beef to pita mixture, and mix until thoroughly combined. Divide into 6 sections. Roll each section into a ball and flatten into a patty about ½ inch thick.

Heat oil in a large skillet over medium-high heat. Add patties and cook until well browned, approximately 3-4 minutes. Turn and cook until second side is also well browned. Drain on paper towels.

Put one beef patty in each warmed pita. Add **Dill** sauce and top with **lettuce**, cucumbers, tomatoes, onion, olives, and feta cheese.

Beef Sirloin/Tenderloin Stroganoff with Dill

(4 servings)

16 ounces extra-wide egg noodles

4 tbsp butter (divided)

2 pounds beef sirloin or tenderloin, trimmed and cut into thin strips (freezing, approximately 15 minutes, makes slicing easier).

2 tbsp extra-virgin olive oil (divided)

Salt, to taste

Garlic powder, to taste

12 ounces **mushrooms**, sliced thick

½ to ⅓ cup red onion, diced

2 tbsp brandy (optional)

4 cups beef stock, reduced by half to two cups or 2 bouillon cubes dissolved in 2 cups water

1 tbsp cornstarch

½ cup water

1 cup sour cream (or to taste)

2 tsp dried **Dill** weed

Cook noodles per package instructions. Drain. Add 2 tbsp butter and keep warm.

Brown beef in 1 tbsp butter and 1 tbsp olive oil over high heat. Season with salt and **Garlic** powder. Remove meat from skillet and drain fat.

In skillet, heat 1 tbsp butter and 1 tbsp olive oil. Add **mushrooms** and onion, and sauté until golden brown.

Return beef to skillet with **mushrooms** and onion. Add brandy and reduced beef stock or bouillon cubes in water. Bring to a simmer.

In a small bowl, whisk cornstarch and water. Add to broth. Simmer for a few minutes until broth has thickened.

Add sour cream and **Dill**. Taste and adjust seasonings if needed.

Serve over warm buttered noodles.

Note: For a medium consistency, use 1 tbsp of cornstarch to thicken every 2 cups of water or stock. If sauce is NOT thick enough, add more cornstarch mixed with sauce in a cup, and then stirred into the mixture. If sauce is too thick, slowly add a little water until sauce is desired consistency.

Meatballs with Dill Dressing

(24 meatballs)

- 1 pound ground beef
- ½ cup bread crumbs
- 1 egg
- ½ small onion, finely chopped
- ½ tsp salt
- 1 tsp dried **Dill** weed
- 1 tsp **Garlic** powder
- 1 tsp onion powder
- ½ tsp dried **basil**
- 1 tsp ground black pepper, divided
- ½ cup ketchup
- ¾ cup tomato puree
- 2 tbsp cider vinegar
- 1 cup cola soda
- 1 onion, chopped
- 1 green bell pepper, chopped
- 1 tsp spice seasoning
- 1 tbsp Worcestershire sauce

Preheat oven to 375 degrees.

In a large bowl, mix together the ground beef, bread crumbs, egg, onion, salt, and **Dill**, **Garlic** powder, onion powder, **basil**, and ½ tsp black pepper until well blended. Let stand for 5 minutes.

Shape into approximately 24 meatballs. Place on baking sheet.

Bake for 30 minutes, turning meatballs over after 15 minutes. When done, remove meatballs from the baking sheet and place in slow cooker.

Combine ketchup, tomato puree, cider vinegar, cola, onion, bell pepper, spice seasoning, ½ tsp black pepper, and Worcestershire sauce. Pour over meatballs in slow cooker.

Cover and cook on high for 1 hour or low for 3-4 hours.

Serve with green salad.

Reuben Sandwich

(1 serving; Frank Nice recipe)

2 tbsp nonfat Thousand Island dressing

2 slices **Dill** or rye bread, lightly toasted

1 ounce pastrami or turkey pastrami

¼ cup sauerkraut, well drained

⅛ cup mozzarella cheese, shredded

1 tbsp mustard

Cooking spray, as needed

1 serving **Dill** pickles

1 serving potato chips

Spread Thousand Island dressing on 1 slice of bread and top with pastrami, sauerkraut, and cheese.

Spread mustard on second slice of bread and put on top (mustard side down) of cheese.

Heat until cheese melts in a nonstick pan, using cooking spray, if needed.

Cut in 2 and serve with **Dill** pickles and potato chips.

Salmon with Mustard Dill Sauce

(8 servings)

3 - 3½ pounds salmon, center cut piece, boned, cleaned, and scaled

1 large bunch **Dill**, washed and patted dry

¼ cup coarse salt

¼ cup granulated sugar

2 tbsp white peppercorns, crushed

1 cup Aquavit or Snaps

4 tbsp prepared dark mustard, highly seasoned

1 tsp dry mustard powder

3 tbsp sugar

2 tbsp white vinegar

⅓ cup vegetable oil

3 tbsp fresh **Dill**, chopped

1 onion, chopped

In a 9 by 13-inch dish, place salmon, skin side down. Top with ⅔ of fresh **Dill**.

Combine salt, sugar and pepper. Sprinkle over fish.

Pour ½ cup Aquavit or Snaps on salmon. Turn salmon skin side up, stacked large end to skinny end.

Place rest of **Dill** on top of salmon. Pour remainder of Aquavit or Snaps over salmon.

Lay a sheet of foil on top of fish. Then, place a tray weighted down with approximately 5 pounds of cans, bricks, or other items on top of salmon. (Be sure tray is smaller than pan and that the weights rest directly over salmon.)

Refrigerate salmon for a minimum of 48 hours or up to 3 days, basting and turning every 12 hours. Separate layers and baste between and over top of salmon.

Combine mustard, mustard powder, sugar, vinegar, oil, and 3 tbsp fresh **Dill** to make sauce. Refrigerate.

To serve, wipe off brine and remove **Dill**. Slice salmon diagonally, as thinly as possible, with a very sharp, thin-bladed knife.

Top with Mustard **Dill** Sauce and chopped onion.

Sides

Creamed Pumpkin with Dill

(8 servings)

Vegetable oil

1 onion, chopped

Salt, to taste

1 tsp ground red cayenne pepper

2-3 pound **pumpkin**, grated

10 ounces sweet cream

¼ cup flour

1 handful fresh **Dill**, chopped

2 tsp vinegar, to taste

1 tsp sugar, to taste

Heat oil. Sauté onion until translucent; then add salt and cayenne pepper.

Add grated **pumpkin**. Sauté until **pumpkin** is tender. Add a little water, if needed.

Mix cream with flour and **Dill**. Add mixture to **pumpkin** and bring to a boil.

Add vinegar, sugar, and salt to achieve a sweet and sour taste.

Serve the **pumpkin** as a side dish with sausages, boiled potatoes, and/or fried eggs.

Potatoes Gratin with Dill

(8 servings)

12 russet potatoes, peeled and cut into ⅛-inch thick slices (divided)

1½ tsp dried **Dill** weed (divided)

3 cups grated Swiss or cheddar cheese (divided)

1⅓ cups whipping cream

1⅓ cups **chicken broth**

¼ cup Dijon mustard

1 tbsp butter

Preheat oven to 400 degrees. Butter a 13 x 9 x 2-inch baking dish.

Layer ⅓ of the potatoes in baking dish, overlapping edges. Season with salt and pepper. Sprinkle with ½ tsp **Dill** and 1 cup cheese. Repeat layers twice, using ⅓ of potatoes, ½ tsp **Dill**, and 1 cup cheese for each layer.

Whisk cream, broth, and mustard in a bowl. Pour over potatoes.

Bake for 1 hour.

Cool 10 minutes before serving.

Fennel

Fennel tastes like licorice. Both **fennel** seeds and bulbs are used. It has the potential to cause allergic reactions and dermatitis.

Fennel (Foeniculi fructus)

Type: Major galactogogue

Medicinal Dose: 0.1 mL to 0.6 mL of oil (equal to 100 mg to 600 mg) daily

Other Uses: For gastrointestinal disorders and as an expectorant

Caution: Fennel may cause allergic reaction and dermatitis.

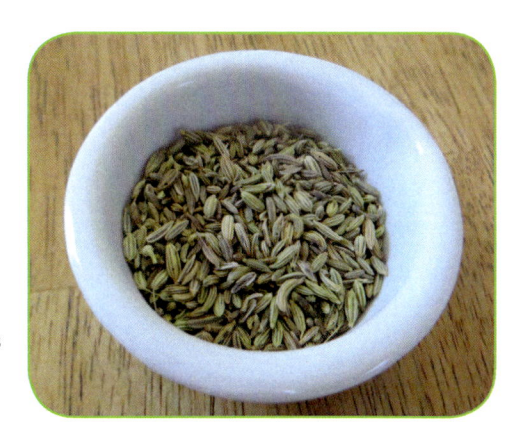

Appetizers

Fennel Fritters

(12 fritters)

2 eggs

¼ cup flour

1 tsp baking powder

½ cup cool water

½ cup grated Parmesan-Romano cheese

¼ tsp salt, plus salt to sprinkle (if necessary)

Freshly ground black pepper, to taste

2 cups canola oil

1 **Fennel** bulb, cut into strips

In a medium-sized bowl, combine eggs, flour, baking powder, water, cheese, salt, and pepper.

Cover and let sit in refrigerator for at least two hours.

In a tall-sided, heavy-bottomed pot, heat oil to 350 degrees.

Remove batter from refrigerator and stir in **Fennel**.

Drop batter by tablespoonfuls into warm oil and fry until crisp. Drain fritters on paper towels.

Serve with your favorite condiment or sauce.

Meatballs with Fennel Sauce

(8 servings)

Olive oil

1 (10-ounce) package frozen chopped **spinach**, thawed

1¼ pounds ground beef

2 eggs

2 cups cooked **rice**

½ cup grated Romano cheese

1 cup shredded mozzarella cheese

¼ tsp ground nutmeg

½ tsp salt

½ tsp fresh ground black pepper

½ tsp red pepper flakes

Fennel sauce (recipe below)

Preheat oven to 400 degrees.

In a large bowl, mix all ingredients together. Form into small balls.

Place on baking sheet and bake for 20-25 minutes, until inside is no longer pink and outside is golden brown.

To serve, top with **Fennel** sauce and additional grated cheese if desired.

Fennel Sauce

Olive oil

2 stalks celery, chopped

¼ head fresh **Fennel**, chopped

4 **Garlic** cloves, chopped

½ cup sliced marinated sweet peppers plus 3 tbsp marinade

3 tbsp raisins

¼ lemon plus squeezed juice

1 (29-ounce) can of crushed tomatoes

2 dashes fresh ground black pepper

2 dashes coarse salt

2 dashes red pepper flakes

1 pinch sugar

Heat a large frying pan with a drizzle of olive oil.

Add celery, **Fennel**, **Garlic**, marinated peppers, and raisins. Add lemon juice and piece of lemon. Sauté until celery is tender.

Add crushed tomatoes, pepper, salt, red pepper flakes, and sugar.

Let simmer, approximately 10-15 minutes.

Bread

Fennel Blue Cheese Flatbread

(1 flatbread)

1½ cups warm water

1 tsp yeast

1 tsp salt

5 cups flour

3 tbsp olive oil, plus additional oil

1 **Fennel** bulb, washed

2 **Garlic** cloves, minced

2 tbsp Greek seasoning (recipe below)

1 (14½-ounce) can petite diced tomatoes, drained

4 ounces blue cheese, crumbled

Preheat oven to 500 degrees.

Mix hot water with yeast; set aside.

In a stand mixer on low, combine salt and flour, and slowly drizzle in 3 tbsp oil. Add water/yeast mixture and continue mixing until a ball forms. Move to a bowl coated with olive oil; cover and refrigerate.

Remove stalks from **Fennel** bulb and throw away, but keep fronds (thin, small strands on top). Slice bulb as thin as possible.

Drizzle olive oil in a large sauté pan over medium-high heat. Add **Garlic**, stir for a few seconds, and then add **Fennel** slices. Stir and combine with olive oil and reduce heat. Sauté until caramelized, approximately 10 minutes. Remove from heat.

Generously coat a pizza size stone (or baking sheet) with olive oil.

Take dough out of refrigerator and cut in half. Save rest for later uses. Spread out dough to cover stone or baking sheet.

Drizzle with olive oil and then sprinkle evenly with Greek seasoning. Layer tomatoes, **Fennel** bulb, and Bleu cheese on top.

Bake for 15-20 minutes, until cheese starts to brown.

Slice into squares and top with **Fennel** fronds.

Greek Seasoning

1½ tsp dried oregano

1 tsp dried mint

½ tsp dried **basil**

½ tsp dried marjoram

½ tsp dried minced onion

½ tsp dried minced **Garlic**

In a small bowl, combine all ingredients.

Store in airtight container in a cool, dry place for up to six months.

Fennel Tea Biscuits

(18 biscuits)

1 tbsp **Fennel** seed, crushed

2 tbsp boiling water

¾ cup butter, softened

²/₃ cup packed brown sugar

1 egg

2 cups flour

½ tsp baking soda

Confectioners' sugar, as needed for rolling

Preheat oven to 350 degrees.

In a small bowl, soak **Fennel** seeds in boiling water. Set aside.

In a large bowl, cream butter and brown sugar until light and fluffy. Beat in egg.

Drain **Fennel** seeds. Add to creamed mixture.

Combine flour and baking soda. Gradually add to creamed mixture. Mix well.

Roll into 1-inch balls. Place 2 inches apart onto ungreased baking sheets.

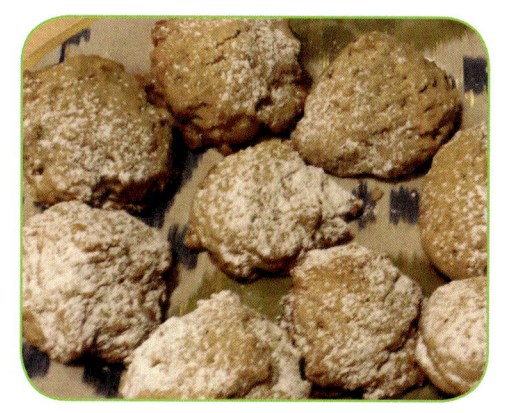

Bake for 10-12 minutes, or until lightly browned.

Roll warm cookies into confectioners' sugar. Cool on wire racks.

Salads

Beet Fennel Salad

(2 servings)

2 large **beets**, peeled and sliced

1 large **Fennel** bulb, thinly sliced

Olive oil

Tony Cachere seasoning, to taste (optional)

Salt, to taste (optional)

Ground black pepper, to taste (optional)

1 large orange, sectioned and sections halved

Feta cheese as garnish

Candied pecans or walnuts as garnish (optional)

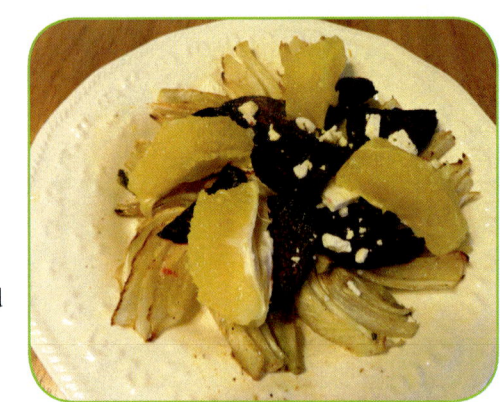

Preheat oven to 400 degrees. Place sliced **beets** on baking sheet. Drizzle with olive oil and seasonings. On another baking sheet placed sliced **Fennel**. Drizzle with olive oil and seasonings. (Do not combine **beets** and **Fennel** because **beets** bleed and will color **Fennel**.) Bake 20 minutes or until **beets** are tender.

When **beets** and **Fennel** are done, layer **Fennel**, **beets**, and oranges on a platter.

Top with feta cheese and candied nuts.

Fennel Cumin Flank Steak Salad

(4 servings)

1 tsp whole **Fennel** seeds

1 tsp whole **cumin** seeds

1 tsp yellow mustard seeds

1 tsp **Garlic** powder

1½ tsp salt (divided)

1 tsp coarsely ground black pepper (divided)

1¼ pounds flank steak

2 tbsp olive oil

1 tbsp cider vinegar

1 pint cherry tomatoes, halved

2 **Garlic** cloves, minced

1 (5-ounce) package baby arugula

1 green bell pepper, cored and diced

1 avocado, peeled, pitted, and diced

1 (4-ounce) log soft goat cheese

½ cup dried cranberries

Heat grill to medium-high. Using an oil-soaked paper towel held with tongs, oil grill grates.

In spice grinder or mortar and pestle, combine **Fennel** seeds, **cumin** seeds, mustard seeds, **Garlic** powder, 1 tsp salt, and ½ tsp pepper. Grind well; then rub mixture over both sides of flank steak.

Grill steak for 4-5 minutes per side for medium-rare. Transfer to a cutting board and let rest for 5 minutes.

In a medium bowl, whisk together olive oil, cider vinegar, ½ tsp salt, and ½ tsp pepper. Add tomatoes and **Garlic**, toss well, and set aside.

Divide arugula among 4 serving plates. Top with bell pepper and avocado. Crumble ¼ goat cheese over each plate of arugula; then, sprinkle with dried cranberries.

Thinly slice steak against the grain; then, heap ¼ of steak on top of each salad.

Spoon ¼ of tomatoes, as well as any liquid in bowl, over each salad.

Serve.

Mushroom Fennel Salad

(4-6 servings)

¼ cup fresh lemon juice

1 lemon zest (colored part of peel)

2 tbsp mayonnaise

2 tsp honey

1 tsp coarse salt

¼ tsp freshly ground black pepper

¼ cup fresh **basil** leaves

½ cup olive oil

1 pound cremini or baby bell or baby Portobello **mushrooms**, brushed

3 tbsp canola oil

Salt, to taste

Freshly ground black pepper, to taste

1 large **Fennel** bulb, trimmed and cut into ⅛-inch thick slices

1 lemon, cut in half and grilled, for garnish

Combine lemon juice and zest, mayonnaise, honey, salt, pepper, **basil**, and olive oil in a blender and blend until smooth to make vinaigrette dressing. (Can be made 60 minutes in advance and refrigerated.)

Heat grill to high.

Place **mushrooms** in a large bowl. Add olive oil, salt, and pepper, and toss to coat. Skewer **mushrooms**, 4 on a skewer.

Place **mushrooms** on grill, until golden brown and slightly charred, approximately 4-5 minutes. Turn over and continue grilling until just cooked through, approximately 3-4 minutes longer. Remove from grill to a cutting board and cut in quarters.

Place **Fennel** in a large bowl, add half of vinaigrette, and toss to combine. Season with salt and pepper.

Top with **mushrooms** and drizzle with more of vinaigrette.

Garnish salad with lemon and serve.

Soups

Potato Fennel Soup

(4 servings)

3 medium **Fennel** bulbs, trimmed, quartered, and cored

1 tbsp butter

1 tbsp olive oil

3 scallions (spring onions), trimmed and sliced

4 cups vegetable stock (divided)

1 large potato, peeled and cubed

Ground black pepper, to taste

Slice **Fennel** into medium-size pieces and keep feathery **Fennel** fronds.

Heat butter and olive oil together in a medium pot over medium-low heat.

Add sliced **Fennel**, scallions, and 1 cup stock. Cover and simmer gently for 15 minutes, until **Fennel** is soft and translucent.

Add potato and remaining 3 cups stock and bring to a boil. Reduce heat to medium-low and simmer gently for 25 minutes or until potato is very soft and cooked through.

Gently mash vegetables with a potato masher or the back of a wooden spoon until soup is thick and chunky (do NOT puree the mixture). Add a small amount of water if mixture becomes too thick.

Season with pepper.

Set aside for 5 minutes before serving to allow flavors to develop.

Entrees

Chicken Pot Pie with Mushrooms and Fennel

(6 servings)

16 baby **carrots** with tops, peeled and trimmed with ½ inch of the tops intact

2 tbsp olive oil

4 ¾ tsp salt, plus additional to taste (divided)

3 pounds (approximately 4 medium) russet potatoes, peeled and quartered

1½ pounds bone-in, skin-on chicken thighs

¼ tsp freshly ground black pepper

2 tbsp olive oil

2 tbsp flour

1½ cups **chicken broth**

2 cups **mushrooms**, sliced

1½ cups small **Fennel** bulb, diced

1 cup small **carrot**, diced

1 cup fresh pearl onions, peeled, or frozen pearl onions, thawed

2 tbsp Dijon mustard

8 tbsp butter, unsalted (divided)

2 tbsp fresh chives, thinly sliced

⅔ cup whole milk (divided)

Preheat oven to 425 degrees. Place baby **carrots** on a small rimmed baking sheet. Drizzle with oil and season with ¼ tsp salt. Roast **carrots** until tender and lightly browned, approximately 20-25 minutes. Keep warm in oven.

Put potatoes in a 4-quart saucepan; add enough water to cover and 4 tsp salt. Cover and bring to a boil over high heat. Cook until tender when pierced with a fork, approximately 12-15 minutes. Drain well.

Season chicken with ½ tsp salt and ¼ tsp pepper.

Heat oil in large skillet over medium-high heat. Cook chicken, flipping once, until lightly browned, approximately 10 minutes. Transfer chicken to a plate.

Reduce heat to medium and whisk flour into the fat in skillet. Cook while whisking for 1 minute. Gradually whisk in **chicken broth** and bring to a simmer.

Return chicken to skillet, reduce heat to medium-low, cover, and simmer gently, turning once, until chicken is very tender, approximately 15 minutes. Transfer chicken to a clean plate and let cool briefly.

Stir **mushrooms**, **Fennel**, diced **carrots**, and onions into sauce. Cover and simmer until tender, approximately 5-6 minutes. Stir in mustard and 2 tbsp butter.

When chicken is cool enough to handle, pull meat from bones, shred into bite-size pieces (discard skin and bones), and add to sauce. Season with salt and pepper.

When potatoes are ready, heat milk in a small saucepan over medium heat until steaming, approximately 2 minutes.

With an electric hand mixer on medium-low speed, beat potatoes until broken up, approximately 1-2 minutes. Add 6 tbsp butter and ½ cup of hot milk. Beat on high speed, scraping sides and bottom of the occasionally, until fluffy, approximately 1-2 minutes (potatoes should be fairly stiff). Add remaining milk, if needed. Season with salt and pepper.

To serve, put warm, whipped potatoes into a pastry bag. Pipe potatoes to form "bowls" on each of 6 plates; bowls should be approximately 3 inches in diameter and approximately 2½ inches tall. If you do not have a pastry bag, line individual bowls with whipped potatoes.

Spoon chicken stew into bowls and garnish with roasted baby **carrots** and chives.

Fennel Stuffed Sea Bass with Broccoli

(3 servings)

1 tbsp olive oil

1 **Fennel** bulb, sliced into wide strips

2 **Garlic** cloves, chopped

¼ cup white wine

¼ cup water

¼ tsp salt

2 heads broccoli, divided into florets

1 tbsp olive oil

1 tsp cracked black pepper

1 serving **basil**, chopped, to taste

1 bunch **Dill**, chopped, to taste

1 pinch salt

3 sea bass, cleaned

Preheat oven to 350 degrees.

Heat olive oil. Add **Fennel** and sauté for 5 minutes. Add **Garlic**, stir fry for 1 minute.

Stir in wine, water, and salt. Reduce heat and simmer, half-covered, for 15 minutes or until **Fennel** is tender and turns golden brown. Set aside to cool.

Microwave broccoli in a small amount of water for 6 minutes or blanch briefly in boiling water. Broccoli must remain firm, but NOT hard. Drain and place onto a baking tray. Lightly season with salt.

Mix olive oil, black pepper, **basil**, **Dill**, and salt to make marinade.

Pat dry each sea bass, inside and out, with paper towels. Make three diagonal cuts in one side of fish down to bone. Stuff cuts and smear marinade over fish.

Fill cavity of each bass with stewed **Fennel**.

Gently transfer fish onto broccoli in baking tray and bake in an oven,

Mussels in Fennel Sauce

(4 servings)

⅓ cup extra-virgin olive oil

1 cup fresh **Fennel**, thinly sliced

½ cup shallots, thinly sliced

⅓ cup **Garlic**, finely chopped

1 cup dry white wine

2 ounces fresh lemon juice

1 tsp **Coriander seeds**

1 tsp **Anise** seeds

2 pounds mussels, scrubbed and beards removed

2 tbsp unsalted butter, cut into 1/4-inch pieces

¼ cup **Fennel** fronds

¼ cup fresh **basil**, chiffonade (roll leaves lengthwise, slice across, and fluff)

In a large sauté pan or Dutch oven, heat olive oil over medium heat. When oil is hot, add **Fennel**, shallots, and **garlic**. Cook, stirring occasionally, until soft and translucent.

Stir in white wine, lemon juice, **Coriander seeds**, and **Anise** seeds. Bring to a boil.

Add cleaned mussels and cover. Cook over medium heat until all mussels have opened, approximately 3-4 minutes.

Add butter, **Fennel** fronds, and fresh **basil**. Mix well. Cook until butter melts.

Serve.

Oriental Chicken Stir Fry

(4 servings)

1 tbsp vegetable oil

6 ounces boneless chicken breast, cut in chunks

1 cup sliced celery

2 cups broccoli florets

⅔ cup red bell pepper, minced

3 green onions, diagonally sliced

1 **Garlic** clove, chopped

2 cups **mushrooms**, sliced

1 **Fennel** bulb, cut into thin strips

½ cup **chicken broth**

1 tbsp cornstarch

2 tsp soy sauce

½ tsp ground **Ginger**

Heat oil over high heat. Add chicken; cook for 3 minutes stirring constantly.

Add celery, broccoli, red pepper, onions, and **Garlic**. Cover and steam for 5 minutes.

Add **mushrooms** and **Fennel**; cover and steam for 2 minutes.

Combine **chicken broth**, cornstarch, soy sauce, and **Ginger**; pour over chicken mix.

Stir-fry for 1 minute or until sauce thickens.

Seared Chicken with Mashed Fennel

(2 servings)

1 **Garlic** bulb, peeled and chopped

2 onions, chopped

4 tbsp olive oil

6 ounces chicken breast

Salt, to taste

Ground black pepper, to taste

5 ounces light cream

1 tbsp almond powder

½ cup **Fennel** bulb, boiled and mashed

1 cup crispy leeks (recipe below)

Heat olive oil in sauté or fry pan Sauté **Garlic** and onions until onions are translucent.

Add chicken, salt, and pepper.

Mix cream with almond powder. Pour over chicken. Cook until chicken is tender.

Serve with mashed **Fennel** and crispy leeks.

Crispy Leeks

   2 leeks

   ¼ cup vegetable oil

   Coarse salt, to taste

Trim leeks of all green parts. Cut them in half lengthwise. Holding each half together, wash all grit away under cold water. Pat dry with paper towels.

Lay each half, cut side down, on a cutting board and slice lengthwise into fine, thin strips. Again pat dry with paper towel.

Heat oil in nonstick pan, add the leeks, and fry for approximately 3 minutes or until golden and crisp. Remove to paper towels and allow to drain well. Season to taste with salt.

When reheating, lay in single layer.

Slow Roasted Pork with Fennel, Tomatoes, and Olives

   (12 servings)

   1 (5 pound) pork shoulder, cut into 2-inch cubes

   Salt, to taste

   Freshly ground black pepper, to taste

   5-8 tbsp extra virgin olive oil, plus more for drizzling

   2 medium yellow onions, peeled and sliced into ¼ inch wedges

   8 large **Garlic** cloves, peeled and trimmed

   1 large **Fennel** bulb, washed and cut into ¼ inch wedges

   1 cup chardonnay or other white wine

   1 (15-ounce) can whole peeled tomatoes with juice

   1 cup pitted and sliced olives

2 bay leaves, fresh or dried

1 tbsp **Fennel** seeds

Preheat oven to 350 degrees.

Season pork with salt and pepper.

Heat 2 tbsp olive oil in a large braising pan over medium-high heat until sizzling.

Add 1 layer of pork to pan. Sear meat until golden brown and crisp on all sides; then, remove to a large plate or bowl. Cook pork in batches, adding more olive oil as needed, until all pork is cooked.

Add 2 tbsp of olive oil to pan. Add onions, **Garlic**, and **Fennel**, and sauté until wilted, approximately 15 minutes.

Add white wine and reduce by half, approximately 5 minutes.

Add tomatoes, olives, bay leaves, and **Fennel** seed, and stir.

Add meat back to pan and place in oven, uncovered.

Roast until juices are thick and meat is tender, approximately 2-3 hours. Turn meat over after 60 minutes. Add water, approximately 1 cup at a time, if juices evaporate before meat is tender. Season with salt and pepper.

To serve, remove bay leaves and spoon pork and vegetables into flat bowls, with some olives and juice. Serve flat bread on the side.

Sides

Roasted Butternut Squash and Fennel

(4 servings)

1 butternut squash, approximately 2½ pounds, peeled, halved lengthwise, seeded, and chopped

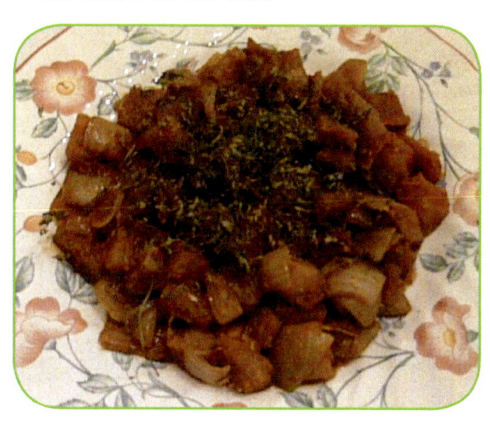

2 Granny Smith apples, peeled, cored, and chopped

2 **Fennel** bulbs, halved lengthwise, cored, and chopped, plus 2 tbsp **Fennel** fronds

½ cup dried cranberries

¼ cup olive oil

1½ tsp salt

½ tsp freshly ground pepper

Preheat oven to 400 degrees.

Toss squash, apples, **Fennel** bulb and fronds, cranberries, oil, salt, and pepper in large bowl until well coated.

Arrange squash mixture in a single layer on a baking sheet.

Roast until vegetables are tender and lightly browned, approximately 15-20 minutes.

Fenugreek

Fenugreek is probably the most used herbal galactogogue. Mothers who are allergic to legumes, especially peanuts, may be allergic to **Fenugreek**.

Fenugreek (Foenugraeci semen)

Type: Major galactogogue

Medicinal Dose: Orally, 6 grams in capsule form daily; externally to treat inflammation, 50 grams in 8 ounces of water

Other Uses: To stimulate appetite, externally to control inflammation

Caution: Fenugreek may cause nausea and vomiting in mother and diarrhea in baby; may increase asthma symptoms or lower glucose levels in mother; may cause skin reactions with external use (avoid nipple area); may cause "maple syrup" smell in mother's and/or baby's urine and/or sweat; do not use if allergic to peanuts and/or legumes.

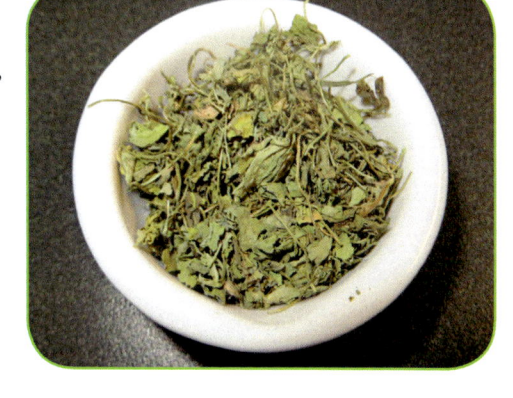

Beverages

Fenugreek Tea

(1 serving; herbal remedy recipe)

1 cup water

1 tbsp **Fenugreek** seeds (do NOT grind)

Honey, to taste

Bring water to boil.

Add **Fenugreek** seeds and boil for 5 minutes.

Remove from heat and steep for 10-15 minutes.

Pour **Fenugreek** tea into a cup through a strainer to remove seeds. Sweeten with honey if desired.

Drink immediately or store in refrigerator to drink later.

Breads

Fenugreek Flatbread

(1 flatbread)

1-1½ cups wheat flour

2 crushed green chilies

1½ tsp red chili powder

½ tsp **turmeric** powder

1 tsp **Coriander** powder

1 tsp **cumin** powder

1 tbsp **Ginger**

1 tsp **Garlic** paste

1 tsp **Caraway** seed

½ bunch **Fenugreek** leaves

Salt, to taste

Vegetable oil, to knead

Water, to knead

Mix flour, spices, and **Fenugreek** leaves in a bowl with enough water and oil to knead into dough.

Set aside for 15 minutes or more. Then roll out and brush each side with oil.

Cook in a frying pan until both sides are crispy and golden brown (kind of like potato pancakes).

Serve warm with chutney.

Condiments

Jamaican Curry Powder

(1 container)

2 tbsp **Coriander seeds**

1 tbsp **cumin** seeds

1 tbsp mustard seeds

1 tbsp **Anise** or **Fennel** seeds

2 tbsp **Fenugreek** seeds

2 tsp whole allspice berries

2½ tbsp ground **turmeric**

In a dry skillet, combine **Coriander seeds**, **cumin** seeds, mustard seeds, **Anise** or **Fennel** seeds, **Fenugreek** seeds, and allspice berries. Toast over medium heat until color of seeds slightly darkens and they become very fragrant, approximately 1 to 2 minutes. Watch closely - it's easy to burn them.

Place seeds in a bowl and let cool to room temperature.

Place seeds in a spice or coffee grinder and grind to a powder.

Put powder in small bowl and add **turmeric**. Mix well.

Store in an airtight container at room temperature.

Tomato Chutney

(1 jar)

1½ pounds red tomatoes, ripe and firm, washed

6 ounces tomato paste

50 **Coriander** leaves (cilantro), chopped

1 tsp salt

1 dash **turmeric**

1 tsp red chili powder

1 tsp mustard seeds

2 tsp **Fenugreek** seeds

2 tsp vegetable oil

3 tsp sugar

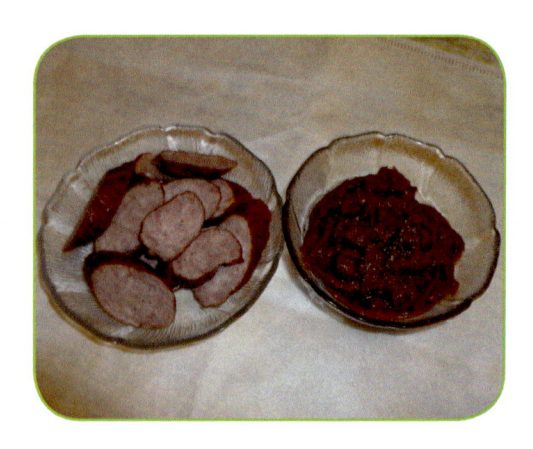

Blanch tomatoes in boiling water for 5-10 minutes.

Cool, peel, and mash tomatoes lightly. Depending on how watery tomatoes are, add up to ½ cup water and puree tomatoes. Strain and discard seeds.

Mix in tomato paste.

Mix in **Coriander** leaves (cilantro).

Combine salt, **turmeric**, red chili powder, mustard seeds, and **Fenugreek** seeds.

Add spice mixture to tomato puree and mix well.

In a deep pan, heat vegetable oil.

Add tomato puree, cover with lid askew, and cook for 30-40 minutes on low heat until all water evaporates, stirring from time to time.

Add sugar and mix well until chutney forms a ketchup-like consistency.

Cool thoroughly and store in an airtight glass jar.

Soups

Butternut Squash Soup

(8 servings)

3 pounds butternut squash, peeled, seeded, and cut in 1-inch squares

1 tbsp curry paste

Salt, to taste

Ground black pepper, to taste

1 tsp **Coriander seeds**

2 tsp **Fenugreek** seeds

1 tsp **Fennel** seeds

1 tsp red pepper flakes or powder

1 tsp **cumin**

1 tsp **turmeric** powder

1 tbsp **Ginger**

½ tsp cinnamon

¼ tsp clove

3 tbsp olive oil

2 medium onions, chopped

1 **Garlic** clove, minced

3 cups water

3 cups tomato juice

24 ounces **coconut** milk

3 tbsp brown sugar (or to taste)

½ bunch **spinach**, chopped

Cooking oil spray, as needed

Preheat oven to 375 degrees.

Put squash and curry paste in a large freezer bag, shaking vigorously until well coated. Season lightly with salt and pepper.

Bake in a flat pan (sprayed with cooking oil) for 30 minutes.

Grind **Coriander seeds**, **Fenugreek** seeds, and **Fennel** seeds into a powder. Mix with red pepper flakes, **cumin**, **turmeric**, **Ginger**, cinnamon, and cloves.

In a large pot, add olive oil, onions, and **Garlic**, and cook until transparent. Add spice mix and cook on medium-low for approximately 1 minute, stirring constantly. Do NOT burn spices.

Add baked squash. Cover with water and tomato juice, and bring to a simmer. Simmer for 30 minutes.

Stir in **coconut** milk.

Puree ingredients with emersion blender until smooth. Bring to a simmer.

Add brown sugar and chopped **spinach**, and simmer until **spinach** is soft.

Season with salt and pepper.

Entrees

Asian Crusted Salmon

(4 servings)

1 tsp **cumin** seeds

1 tsp black mustard seeds

1 tsp **Fennel** seeds

¼ tsp **Fenugreek** seeds

¼ tsp **Garlic** powder

½ tsp **Ginger** powder

1 tbsp paprika

1½ tsp salt

4 (6-ounce) salmon fillets, skin removed

½ tbsp vegetable oil

12 lemon wedges, for garnish

Grind all seeds in an electric spice or coffee grinder (or with a mortar and pestle).

Mix ground spices with **Garlic**, **Ginger**, paprika, and salt in a small bowl.

Dry salmon fillets and rub spice mixture on both sides of each fillet. Let sit for 30 minutes or more.

Heat oil in a large sauté pan over highest possible heat. When oil is smoking, add salmon fillets and cook on 1 side for 2 minutes; then flip and cook on other side for 2 more minutes.

Remove from pan and serve with lemon wedges for garnish.

Fenugreek Cashew Chicken

(6 servings)

6 chicken legs
8 tbsp plain yogurt
4 tsp salt (divided)
4 tbsp vegetable oil
1 dry red chili pepper
2 whole 1-inch cinnamon sticks
1 whole black cardamom
4 whole green cardamoms
6 cloves
6 black peppercorns
1 tsp **cumin** seeds
½ onion, cut lengthwise, thinly
¾ cup onion paste (recipe below)
¼ tsp nutmeg
¼ tsp mace
¾ tsp **turmeric** powder
5 tbsp **Garlic** paste (recipe below)
2 tsp **Ginger** paste (make by mincing fresh **Ginger**)
2 tbsp cashew nut butter (recipe below)
3 tbsp water
1 tsp **cumin** powder
3 tbsp dry **Fenugreek** leaves
1½ tsp red chili powder (optional)
4 fresh red or green chili peppers
3 cups water

Marinate chicken legs with yogurt and 3 tsp salt. Place in refrigerator for at least 5 hours.

In a heavy-bottomed wok or skillet, add vegetable oil and wait until it smokes at medium heat. Add dry red chili, cinnamon sticks, black cardamom, green cardamoms, cloves, black peppercorns, and **cumin** seeds and wait until **cumin** seeds just turn dark brown.

Immediately add onions and sauté until brownish.

Add onion paste, nutmeg, mace, and **turmeric**, and sauté for 2 minutes.

Add **Garlic** paste and **Ginger** paste, along with 1 tsp salt. Sauté until mixture releases oil (takes 7-10 minutes at medium heat).

Add cashew nut butter and 3 tbsp water. Stir and cook at medium heat for 5 minutes.

Add marinated chicken, **cumin** powder, and dried **Fenugreek** leaves. Coat chicken legs evenly in mixture.

Cover with lid and cook over medium heat for 30 minutes. The chicken should acquire a brown tinge.

Add red chili powder (optional), fresh chilies, and 3 cups water and mix.

Replace lid and simmer at lowest heat for 60 minutes (slow-cooking will lead to perfectly succulent chicken legs with all flavors reaching into deepest parts of chicken).

Serve with **rice** or potatoes.

Onion Paste

    1 large (½ pound) onion

    1 cup water

In a small saucepan, combine onion and water and bring to a boil.

Simmer over low heat until onion is just tender, approximately 15 minutes.

Using a slotted spoon, transfer onion to blender and puree.

Can be stored in refrigerator for up to 5 days.

Garlic Paste

    2 **Garlic** cloves, peeled and halved

    ½ cup water

In a blender, puree **Garlic** with water.

Can be refrigerated up to 5 days (may darken but still will be good).

Cashew Nut Butter

    1¼ cups raw cashews, unsalted

    1 tbsp canola or olive oil

½ tbsp orange or lemon juice

¼ tsp salt

In a blender, process cashews until a very fine, almost powdery, meal-like consistency.

Add oil, orange or lemon juice, and blend for 30-60 seconds.

Using rubber spatula, scrape down blender sides, making sure mixture is uniform, with no clumps at the bottom.

Blend 30 seconds. Taste and add more salt and/or oil if needed.

Transfer to airtight container and refrigerate or put in zip lock bag and freeze.

Fried Chicken Liver

(4 servings)

3 medium onions, chopped

1 tsp **cumin** seeds

½ cup vegetable oil

1 pound fresh chicken liver, sliced

1 tbsp vinegar

1 tsp salt

¼ tsp ground black pepper

½ cup water

1 tsp **Fenugreek** seeds

1 tbsp **Coriander seeds**

Brown onions and **cumin** seeds in hot oil.

Add chicken liver and vinegar. Season with salt and black pepper. Stir fry for 10 minutes.

Add water and simmer until water is absorbed.

Add **Fenugreek** seeds and cook for 5 minutes.

Garnish with **Coriander seeds**.

Leftover Turkey/Chicken Curry

(8 servings)

1 pound dried pasta (penne or fusilli work well; use whole wheat, if possible)

3 cups broccoli, diced

2 tbsp butter

1 medium onion, diced

½-inch fresh **Ginger**, grated

2 **Garlic** cloves, minced

2 tbsp flour

2 cups **chicken broth**

2 tsp curry powder (or more if desired)

1 tsp **Fenugreek** powder

Salt, to taste

Ground black pepper, to taste

2 cups leftover turkey or chicken, diced

¼ cup **Coriander seeds**

Cook pasta according to package instructions. Add broccoli the last 4 minutes of cooking. Drain and set aside.

Heat butter in empty pasta pot. Sauté onions until soft, approximately 3-5 minutes.

Add **Ginger** and **Garlic** and cook 30 seconds. Add flour and whisk for 30 seconds.

Add **chicken broth**, a small amount at a time, whisking until incorporated and thickened.

Add curry powder and **Fenugreek** powder.

Add salt and pepper to taste.

Toss in turkey or chicken and heat through.

Add pasta, broccoli, and **Coriander seeds**, and fold in until blended.

Oven Baked Herring

(2 servings)

2 herrings, cleaned
1 tsp red chili powder
¼ tsp **turmeric** powder
⅛ tsp **Fenugreek** powder
Fresh ground black pepper, to taste
Salt, to taste
2 tbsp vegetable oil

Preheat oven to 400 degrees.

Mix chili powder, **turmeric**, **Fenugreek**, pepper and salt. Coat herring with dry powder mix.

Place herring on baking tray lined with aluminum foil.

Splash vegetable oil on top and bake for 15 minutes.

Serve hot with **rice** and salad.

Sides

Deep Purple Potatoes

(8 servings)

1 pound of All Blue potatoes (check local farmers' markets; if not available, use baking potatoes - of course, they will NOT be blue or purple), diced
2 tbsp white vinegar
3 tbsp vegetable oil
1 tsp **Fennel** seeds
1 tsp **cumin** seeds
1 tsp whole brown mustard seed
12 whole **Fenugreek** seeds
3 whole dried red peppers
1½ tsp salt plus to taste

½ tsp **turmeric** powder

1 tbsp lemon juice

Boil potatoes approximately 10 minutes in salted water containing white vinegar. Drain and let cool.

In a skillet, heat vegetable oil. When oil is hot, add **Fennel**, **cumin**, mustard seed, and **Fenugreek**.

When seeds start to darken, add dried red peppers.

When red peppers start to darken, add diced potatoes. Season with salt and **turmeric**.

Turn heat down to medium and stir fry for approximately 15 minutes. Potatoes will turn crispy.

Remove peppers if too hot for taste.

Squeeze lemon juice over potatoes and serve as potato salad.

Desserts

Saint Hildegard Cookies

(18 cookies)

½ cup butter, softened

½ cup honey

1 egg

2 cups flour

1 tbsp baking soda

2 tsp ground cinnamon

½ tsp ground nutmeg

½ tsp ground cloves

½ tbsp ground **Fenugreek**

½ tsp ground cardamom

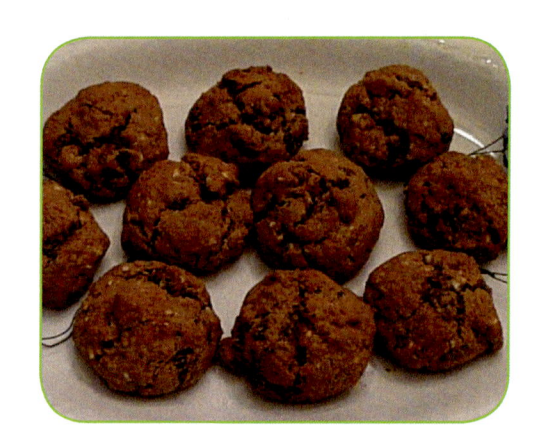

1 cup raisins

½ cup almonds, chopped

1 tbsp **flax seeds** soaked in 3 tbsp water

In a small bowl, cream butter, honey, and egg.

In a large bowl, sift together flour, baking soda, cinnamon, nutmeg, cloves, **Fenugreek**, and cardamom.

Add raisins, almonds, and soaked **flax seeds**.

Add butter mixture to flour mixture and mix well to form dough. Refrigerate until dough is chilled.

When ready to bake, preheat oven to 350 degrees.

Roll chilled dough into small balls, about 1 inch in diameter. Place balls on a cookie sheet. Flatten with a fork.

Put in oven and bake until golden brown, about 12 minutes.

Garlic

Garlic may increase or decrease nursing time. Some babies like the taste of **Garlic** and may drink even more milk. Initially, other babies may be turned off by the smell of **Garlic** in breast milk. These babies may get used to the taste of **Garlic** and return to baseline nursing times.

Garlic (Allii sativi bulbus)

Type: Major galactogogue

Medicinal Dose: 4 grams to 9 grams, in capsule form, daily

Other Uses: For possible positive cardiovascular effects and/or immune system stimulation

Caution: Garlic may decrease nursing time due to odor in breast milk, which some babies may not like.

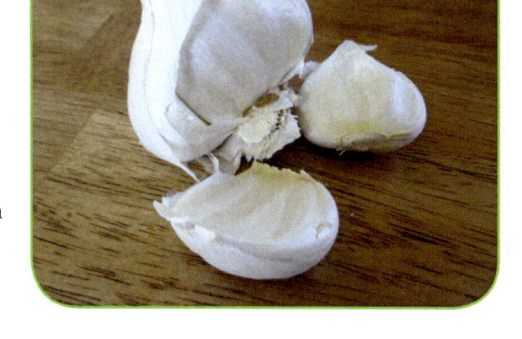

Appetizers

Garlic Hummus

(4-6 servings)

1 (16-ounce) can **chickpeas** (garbanzo beans), drain, reserving ⅓ cup of liquid

1 tbsp tahini (recipe below)

2 tbsp olive oil, plus additional as garnish

3 tbsp lemon juice (divided)

3 **Garlic** cloves, peeled (divided)

¼ tsp salt

Sweet paprika, for garnish

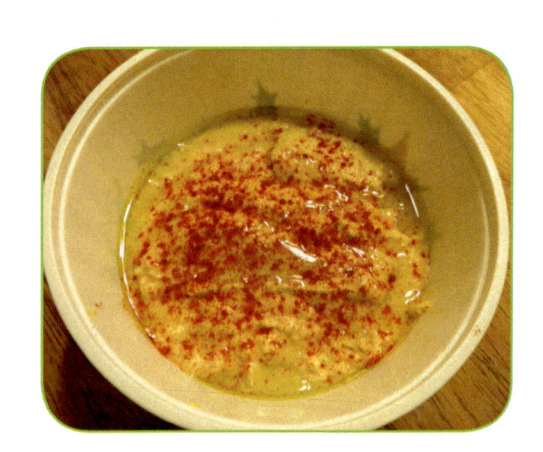

In a food processor or blender, blend **chickpeas**, chickpea liquid, tahini, olive oil, lemon juice, **Garlic** cloves, and salt until smooth. Taste. Add additional lemon juice, **Garlic**, and salt if needed.

Garnish with a dash of olive oil and paprika.

Serve with pita bread, chopped vegetables, and/or your favorite chips.

Tahini

1 cup **sesame seeds**

¼ cup olive oil or vegetable oil

Toast **sesame seeds** in a dry, heavy skillet for 1 to 2 minutes, tossing frequently with a spatula. Do NOT allow to brown. Cool for 20 minutes.

Pour **sesame seeds** into food processor. Add oil and blend for 2 minutes. Oil should be thick, yet pourable. If tahini is not correct consistency, add more oil.

Refrigerate.

Soups

Black Bean Soup

(4 servings)

3 tbsp olive oil

1½ tbsp smoked **cumin**

1 large onion, chopped

2 large **carrots**, chopped

2 ribs celery, chopped

4 **Garlic** cloves, peeled and chopped

3 cans black beans, undrained

1 bay leaf

1 smoked ham hock

2 cups **chicken stock**

Salt, to taste

Ground black pepper, to taste

Tabasco sauce, to taste

1 tbsp fresh lime juice

Sour cream, as topping

Coriander seeds, as topping

Heat olive oil in soup pot. Add **cumin** and cook until fragrant.

Add onions, **carrots**, celery, and **Garlic**, and sauté until golden brown.

Add black beans, bay leaf, ham hock, **chicken stock**, salt, pepper, and Tabasco sauce, and simmer for 30 minutes.

Remove ham hock and bay leaf, and discard. Let soup cool.

Place cooled soup in food processor in batches and puree. Add more **chicken stock** if needed to attain desired consistency. Stir in lime juice.

To serve, top with dollops of sour cream and **Coriander seeds**.

Garlic and Poached Egg Soup

(6 servings)

3 tbsp extra-virgin olive oil

1 **Garlic** bulb, separated into cloves and peeled

2 tsp salt

Freshly ground black pepper, to taste

1 bay leaf

4 **Dill** sprigs

2 quarts water

6 eggs

Dill, chopped, as garnish

Grated Parmesan cheese, as garnish

6 slices Crusty bread

In large saucepan, heat olive oil. Add **Garlic**, salt, pepper, bay leaf, and **Dill** sprigs. Cook until **garlic** is translucent.

Add water. Place over high heat and bring to a boil. Reduce heat to low and simmer for 30 minutes.

Pour through fine-meshed strainer into heatproof bowl, pressing **garlic** to squeeze as much flavor into broth as possible. Discard contents left in strainer.

Let cool. Transfer to a covered container and refrigerate until needed.

To prepare each serving, ladle approximately 1⅓ cups of broth into a saucepan.

Place over medium-low heat and bring to a simmer.

Carefully break an egg for each serving into broth (do NOT break yolk). Poach until white is just set, approximately 1½ minutes (it will continue to cook off the heat).

Transfer each egg to a soup bowl. Pour broth gently over each serving.

Garnish each serving with **Dill** and cheese. Serve with crusty bread.

Nice Polish White Borscht

(Multiple Servings. It is Polish tradition to make enough to feed extended family at Christmas and Easter. The amount made will last for several months stored in the refrigerator with occasional stirring or shaking. If you wish to make less, the recipe can be halved except for the egg. Grandpa Nice, Frank Senior, and Frank Junior developed this recipe.)

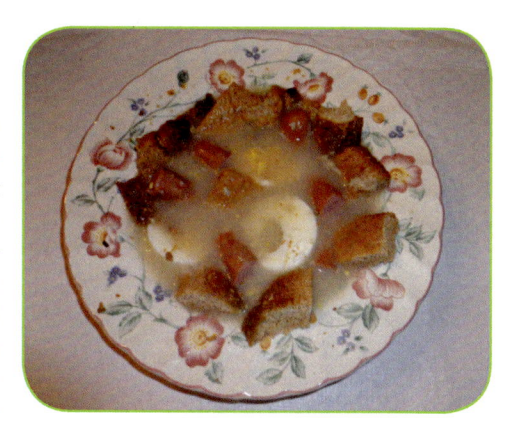

1 pound rye graham (course grain) flour (check on-line)

12 quarts water, divided

4 **Garlic** bulbs, separated into cloves, peeled, and cut into small pieces

2 tbsp salt

1 egg

1 cup milk

½ pound bacon, fried and crushed, or store bought bacon bits (optional)

Vinegar, to taste (optional)

Several days ahead of when you plan to prepare borscht, add flour to 4 quarts water. Mix well. Let set in a warm place to sour, stirring daily until it reaches desired sourness. Stir thoroughly and strain through a fine wire sieve. Freeze flour portion remaining in sieve for use as a starter the next time this recipe is made.

Place **Garlic** pieces in bowl and crush. Add salt and egg. Mix well. Stir in milk and set aside.

Bring 6-8 quarts water (amount will affect final thickness) to a boil. When water is boiling, add strained flour liquid, stirring constantly (or flour will burn on bottom of pot). Continue to stir and bring water back to a boil.

Add **Garlic** mixture, stirring in well.

For extra taste treat, add fried bacon or bacon pieces. If not sour enough, add vinegar to taste.

Place broken bread pieces, pork chunks, ham chunks, kielbasa slices, other favorite meats, hardboiled egg chunks or slices, ground black pepper, or anything else desired into hot borscht.

Leftover borscht can be stored several months in refrigerator. If stored for a long time, stir or shake weekly.

Note: For future batches, unfreeze starter flour and add to initial flour mixture to speed up the souring process.

String Bean Garlic Soup

(4 servings)

> 8 ounces thinly sliced bacon, cut into small strips
>
> 1 onion, finely chopped
>
> 3 **Garlic** cloves, peeled and finely sliced
>
> 1 pound young, **green beans**, cut in half
>
> 1 large **carrot**, thinly sliced
>
> 1 stalk celery, finely chopped
>
> 8 ounces canned diced tomatoes
>
> 1 tbsp tomato paste
>
> 1 generous pinch dried **basil**
>
> 2 cups **chicken stock**
>
> 1 pinch sugar
>
> ¼ tsp ground black pepper
>
> 1 cup small sized pasta
>
> Grated Parmesan cheese, as garnish

Fry bacon with onion until onion is translucent, stirring often.

Add **Garlic** and cook for another 1-2 minutes.

Stir in **green beans**, **carrots**, celery, and tomatoes. Cover and simmer over low heat until vegetables are tender.

Stir in tomato paste and **basil**.

Add **chicken stock**, sugar, and pepper. Bring to a boil, then reduce heat and simmer for 15 minutes.

Add pasta and cook until pasta is firm, but not hard.

To serve, top with Parmesan cheese.

Entrees

Baked Spaghetti Casserole

(8 servings)

1 pound lean ground beef

1 approximately 28-ounce jar or can prepared spaghetti sauce

12 ounces spaghetti

8 ounces cream cheese

1 tsp Italian seasoning

1 **Garlic** clove, peeled and minced

½ cup grated Parmesan cheese

In a skillet, brown ground beef until cooked through. Drain fat. Stir in spaghetti sauce. Set aside.

Cook spaghetti according to directions on package. Drain and place cooked spaghetti in bowl. Add cream cheese, Italian seasoning, and minced **Garlic**. Stir until cream cheese is melted and spaghetti is thoroughly coated.

Preheat oven to 350 degrees. Lightly grease a 9 by 13-inch pan.

Spread small amount of meat sauce in bottom of pan. Put spaghetti on top of sauce and top with remaining meat sauce. Sprinkle Parmesan cheese on top.

Bake for 30 minutes, until bubbly.

BBQ Boneless Chicken Breast

(8 servings)

1 tsp chili powder

1 tsp **Garlic** powder

½ tsp salt

1 tsp brown sugar

1 tsp **curry** powder

1 tsp ground **cumin**

1 tsp **molasses (black strap)**

1 tsp lime juice

1 tbsp olive oil

3 pounds boneless chicken breast

Preheat oven to 350 degrees.

Combine all ingredients, except chicken, in a small bowl, and stir to make a paste.

Place chicken breasts in a baking pan and rub all over with paste.

Bake for 35-40 minutes, depending on how thick chicken breast is. (Do NOT overcook chicken breast, or it will become dry. To check for doneness, cut into thickest part to see if juices run clear.)

Beef Stew

(8 servings)

1 (3-pound) chuck roast, cut in 1½-inch cubes, fat trimmed

Flour, as coating

¼ cup vegetable oil

1½ cups onions, chopped

3-4 **Garlic** cloves, peeled

1 cup dry California red wine

2 cups beef broth

2 bay leaves

4-5 **carrots**, peeled and cut in ¼-inch slices

4 medium red or Yukon gold potatoes

4 medium celery stalks, sliced

1 cup frozen **peas**, thawed

1 (15-ounce) can diced tomatoes

2 tbsp Worcestershire sauce

Salt, to taste

Ground black pepper, to taste

Toss beef cubes with flour (lightly coat). Brown cubes in oil.

Add onions and sauté until lightly browned. Add **Garlic** and cook 30 seconds.

Add wine, broth, and bay leaves. Bring to boil. Cover and simmer on stovetop or place in 350 degree oven for 60 minutes, or until meat is tender.

Add **carrots**, potatoes, and celery. Cook until the vegetables are tender. Add **peas**, tomatoes, and Worchestershire sauce Reheat to original temperature if serving immediately.

Remove and discard bay leaf. Season with salt and pepper.

Note: Stew is best served second day after flavors blend.

Garlic Balsamic Halibut or Sea Bass

(4 servings)

2 tbsp balsamic vinegar

2 tbsp olive oil

2 tsp soy sauce

2 **Garlic** cloves, peeled and minced

Salt, to taste

Fresh ground black pepper, to taste

2 pounds sea bass or halibut steak or fillets

In a small bowl, whisk together vinegar, olive oil, soy sauce, and **Garlic** to make marinade. Add salt and pepper. Taste to adjust seasoning.

Put fish in a zip lock bag and pour in marinade. Turn to coat evenly. Refrigerate for 1-2 hours.

Preheat oven to 425 degrees.

Remove fish from marinade and place in roasting pan. Roast approximately 10 minutes per inch of thickness, until fish is flaky but still moist. Check with fork, if needed.

Cut into serving pieces and serve with juice from pan.

Glazed Pork Chops

(4 servings)

3 tsp plus ¼ tsp black pepper, cracked

4 boneless pork chops, trimmed

2 tbsp honey

2 tbsp soy sauce

1 tbsp balsamic vinegar

½ tsp cornstarch

½ tsp butter, melted

2 **Garlic** cloves, peeled and minced

Fresh chives or green onions, sliced, as garnish

Rub 3 tsp black pepper into one side of pork chops.

Heat nonstick skillet until hot. Add pork chops (pepper side down) and cook approximately 4 minutes or until browned.

Reduce heat to medium, turn pork chops, and cook 6-8 minutes longer. When done, remove skillet from heat, cover pork chops, and set aside.

Mix honey, soy sauce, balsamic vinegar, and cornstarch until smooth to make sauce. Stir in ¼ tsp cracked pepper.

Melt butter in small pan. Add **Garlic** and cook for 30 seconds, stirring.

Stir in honey mixture. Bring to a boil and cook for 1 minute, stirring.

Spoon sauce over pork chops. Sprinkle with fresh chives or green onions.

Lasagna

(8 servings)

1 pound lean ground beef

1 pound ground sausage

1 approximately 28-ounce jar or can prepared spaghetti sauce

1 tbsp minced **Garlic**

2 tbsp extra-virgin olive oil

12 lasagna noodles

2 (8 oz) blocks cream cheese

1 large carton light sour cream

2 approximately 8-ounce bags Italian blend shredded cheese

In a large skillet, brown beef and sausage. Drain fat.

Add spaghetti sauce, **Garlic**, and olive oil. Simmer on low until lasagna is ready to be constructed.

Boil noodles according to package instructions. Drain and set aside.

In a mixing bowl, combine cream cheese and sour cream, and mix well.

Preheat oven to 350 degrees.

In a 9 by 13-inch glass baking dish, begin with a layer of 3 noodles. Spread ¼ of the cream mixture on top of noodles, then ¼ of the meat sauce, and top with ¼ of the shredded cheese. Repeat layers until all noodles have been used.

Bake for 20-30 minutes, until bubbly.

Prime Rib with Horseradish Sauce

(8 servings)

5 pounds prime rib, bone-in

6 **Garlic** cloves, peeled and cut in halves

Favorite steak seasoning, to taste

1 stick butter, melted

1 cup **cherry** or apple juice

½ cup water

¼ cup Worcestershire or steak sauce

Horseradish sauce (recipe below)

Grated Parmesan cheese, as garnish

Using a knife, dig 12 small 1-inch diameter holes uniformly throughout prime rib surface. Push 1 halved **Garlic** clove into each hole. Rub steak seasoning on meat. Tie prime rib with twine at 1-inch intervals.

Put prime rib in baking pan, bone side down, and place smoker at 225-250 degrees (can be smoked using indirect heat on a large grill or in a traditional smoker, using a combination of charcoal and wood or only wood). Close lid and smoke for 60 minutes.

Combine butter, **cherry** or apple juice, water, and Worchestershire or steak sauce. Use to baste or spray prime rib. Repeat basting whenever charcoal or wood is added to fire.

Smoke until meat thermometer inserted into center of prime rib reaches 130 degrees (medium rare with 2 outside slices medium), approximately 4 hours. To insure meat is not overcooked, test every half hour after the meat has been smoking for several hours.

Remove meat from heat, slice bones from meat, make a foil tent to cover beef, and let rest for 30 minutes to maximize flavor. Reserve juice in bottom of pan.

Carve meat. Serve with horseradish sauce and prime rib juice collected from bottom of pan. Garnish with grated Parmesan cheese.

Horseradish Sauce

¼ cup creamy horseradish sauce

2 tbsp cream, sour cream, or mayonnaise

Mix ingredients together and refrigerate until needed.

Yankee Chili

(8 servings)

3 pounds lean chuck roast, diced into ¼-inch pieces (or ground venison with suet)

1 tbsp chili powder (add more, to taste)

3 tbsp **cumin**, ground

3 tbsp oregano, dried

½-1½ tsp cayenne (adjust, to taste)

6 **Garlic** cloves, peeled and minced

1-1½ quarts cold, fresh water (first portion)

1-2 tsp salt

⅓ cup corn meal (coarse, if possible)

⅓ cup cold, fresh water (second portion)

Brown meat. Cook until grease has cooked away.

Add chili powder, **cumin**, oregano, cayenne, and **Garlic**. Mix well.

Add first portion cold, fresh water to just cover meat.

Bring to boil for 1 minute, then turn down heat and simmer for 60-90 minutes. Add salt to taste.

Make paste of corn meal and second portion cold, fresh water, and stir until smooth.

Stir corn meal paste into chili gradually, and simmer another 45 minutes.

Ladle into bowls.

Zucchini Soufflé with Garlic Croutons

(4 servings)

4 ounces sausage

1 **Garlic** clove, peeled and minced

2 tbsp onion, minced

5 eggs, separated

1 cup zucchini, shredded finely

⅓ cup sour or heavy cream

1 tsp Italian herbs

1 cup sharp white cheddar cheese, shredded (divided)

¼ tsp cream of tartar

Garlic croutons (recipe below)

Preheat oven to 375 degrees. Butter and flour a soufflé dish.

In a skillet, sauté crumbled sausage with **Garlic** and onion until sausage is done and onions are translucent. Remove from heat and let cool.

In a large bowl, whisk egg yolks. Stir in zucchini, sour or heavy cream, Italian herbs, ¾ cup cheese, and sausage mixture.

In another large bowl, beat egg whites until foamy; add cream of tartar and beat until stiff glossy peaks form.

Fold ¼ of the egg whites into the egg yolk mixture. Add **Garlic** croutons. Then gently fold this mixture back into remaining egg whites.

Spoon into soufflé dish. Sprinkle with remaining croutons and ¼ cup cheese.

Bake until set and golden brown, approximately 25 minutes. Be careful not to over-bake or soufflé will toughen and dry.

Serve.

Garlic Croutons

1 **Garlic** clove, peeled and minced

1 tbsp olive oil

2 slices sourdough French bread, cut into ½-inch cubes, approximately 1⅓ cups

Preheat oven to 375.

In a bowl, combine **Garlic** and oil. Add bread cubes and toss to coat.

Pour onto cookie sheet, spreading out to make one layer.

Bake 5 minutes or until lightly toasted and golden brown.

Sides

Garlic and Herb Mashed Potatoes

(8 servings; Polish ancestors' recipe)

8-12 red potatoes, scrubbed and cut into quarters (leave skin on)

1 tbsp olive oil

2 **Garlic** cloves, peeled

½ stick butter, room temperature

1 tbsp fresh **Dill**, chopped

1 tbsp fresh green onion, chopped

¼ cup milk, heated to room temperature in microwave just before use

Boil potatoes in large pot of water until tender.

Heat oil in a small skillet and sauté **Garlic** cloves until tender. Remove **Garlic** from oil, pat dry, mash with side of chef's knife (or bottom of heavy jar), and chop as finely as possible.

Drain potatoes, put in large mixing bowl, and mash with potato masher, back of large spoon, or a hand mixer.

Add butter, **Dill**, **Garlic**, and green onion.

Using a large spoon for chunkier potatoes or a hand mixer for creamier potatoes, gradually add milk, blending until desired consistency is reached.

Garlic Quinoa

(4 servings)

2 tsp olive oil or canola oil

1 **Garlic** clove, peeled and chopped

1 cup **quinoa seeds**

2 cups vegetable broth

1 tsp ground black pepper

1 large **carrot**, chopped

1 cup fresh or thawed frozen **peas**

Heat olive oil in a saucepan over medium heat. Add **Garlic** and sauté until translucent.

Lower heat and stir in **quinoa seeds**.

Add vegetable broth, **carrots**, and pepper.

Bring to a boil. Cover, reduce heat to low, and simmer until **carrots** are tender.

Stir in **peas**. Cover and simmer until broth is absorbed, approximately 10 minutes.

Serve.

Sautéed Brussels Sprouts

(6 servings)

2 pounds Brussels sprouts, cut in half

2 **Garlic** cloves, peeled and chopped

¼ cup extra-virgin olive oil

Salt, to taste

Ground black pepper, to taste

Grated Parmesan cheese, as garnish

Boil Brussels sprouts for 10-15 minutes, depending on desired crunchiness. Drain.

Heat olive oil in large sauté pan. Add **Garlic** and sauté over medium heat until golden brown.

Add sprouts and sauté until golden brown, stirring frequently. Season with salt and pepper.

Top with grated Parmesan cheese.

Goat's Rue

This is one section of recipes where the introduction will be longer than the list of recipes. I could only find one recipe for **Goat's rue**. This is probably due to its reputed bitter taste due to its tannin content. Steeping may reduce its bitterness, as well as adding a sweetener. Because of its cost, adding **Goat's rue** to recipes may not be as cost effective as taking the tincture or capsules. This is somewhat unfortunate as **Goat's rue** has the potential to be the herbal galactogogue of choice in the future. The active ingredient, galegin, is related to metformin, which is used to treat Polycystic Ovarian Syndrome (PCOS). Metformin has helped some women to increase milk production. **Goat's rue** and galegin increase milk production 30% or more in goats, sheep, and cows. Why is the herb called **Goat's rue**? Goats and sheep can stuff themselves with **Goat's rue** and go into respiratory depression, as they are very sensitive to galegin. Fortunately, cows and human beings are immune from this bad effect.

Goat's Rue (Galegae officinalis herba)

Type: Major galactogogue

Medicinal Dose: 1 mL to 2 mL of tincture, 2 to 3 times a day; 425 mg capsules 3 to 4 times a day

Other Uses: To lower blood glucose levels

Caution: None.

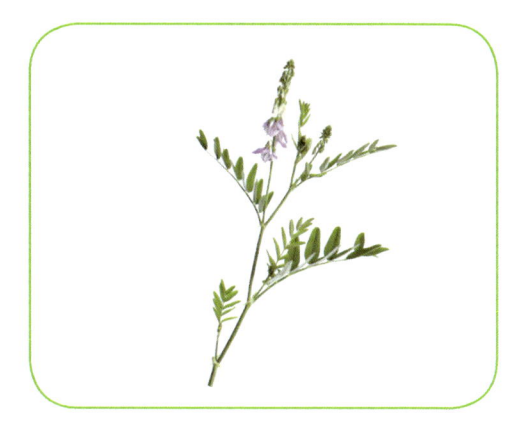

Beverages

Goat's Rue Tea

(2 servings)

    1 tsp dried **Goat's rue** root
    1 pint water

Boil water.
Add dried **Goat's rue** root.
Steep 15-20 minutes.
Strain and drink.

Marshmallow Root

These are not Kraft marshmallows, but you can make the real thing using **Marshmallow Root**.

Marshmallow Root (Althaeae radix)

Type: Minor galactogogue

Medicinal Dose: Two (2) 500 mg capsules 3 times a day; 60 grams daily as tincture or tea

Other Uses: Diuretic

Caution: Marshmallow root rarely may cause allergic reaction.

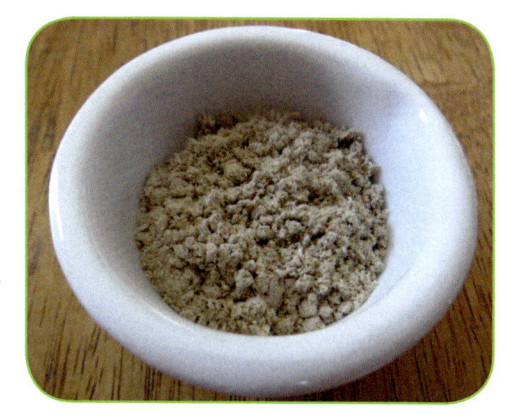

Desserts

Chocolate Mousse with Marshmallow Root Fluff

(2 servings)

Chocolate Layer

1 avocado

2 tbsp carob powder (or 1 tbsp cocoa)

¼ cup plus 1 tbsp **coconut** milk

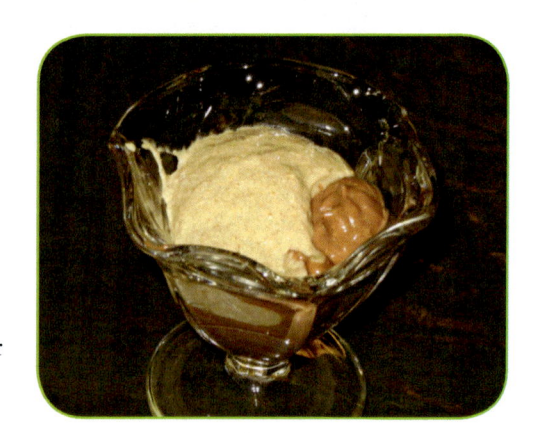

1 tbsp sugar

Marshmallow Layer

⅓ cup full-fat **coconut** milk

1-2 tbsp **Marshmallow Root** powder (depending on desired thickness)

1 tbsp sugar

Blend ingredients listed under chocolate layer in a blender or food processor.

Layer half in bottom of each of two small dessert cups.

Mix together ingredients in marshmallow layer by hand.

Layer half on top of chocolate mousse in each dessert cup.

Refrigerate at least one hour before serving.

Marshmallow Root Marshmallows

(Approximately 50 marshmallows)

½ cup water

½ cup rose water (purchase at natural foods store or make your own like pharmacists do – see recipe below)

1 tbsp **Marshmallow Root** powder

1-2 tbsp **hibiscus** flowers (to make marshmallows pink)

1 packet unflavored gelatin

1 cup honey

1 tsp vanilla extract

1 pinch salt

Bring water and rose water to a boil in a small saucepan. Add **Marshmallow Root** and **hibiscus** flowers, and stir with a whisk. Simmer for 5 minutes, and then refrigerate until cool.

Strain **Marshmallow Root/hibiscus** mixture through a fine mesh sieve. Add enough water to equal a full cup.

Take half of the Marshmallow mixture and place in a medium sized bowl. Add gelatin and mix. Set aside.

Place other half of the mixture in a small saucepan along with honey, vanilla extract, and salt. Bring to a simmer. Place candy thermometer in mixture until it reaches 240 degrees and soft balls form; then remove from heat.

Using a hand mixer, begin to mix **Marshmallow Root**/gelatin mixture on low. Slowly add hot **Marshmallow Root**/honey mixture, while continuing to mix. Once the two mixtures have been combined, continue to whip on high for another 5-10 minutes until fluffy.

Pour mixture into an 8 by 8-inch pan lined with natural parchment paper that has been oiled.

Let sit for a few hours until set up and firm.

Slice with a knife (may be sticky; roll in powdered sugar to make less sticky).

Rose Water

2-3 quarts fresh roses or rose petals

1 portion water, as needed

2-3 trays ice cubes or 1 bag crushed ice

Place a washed clean firebrick in center of large pot (speckled blue canning pots are ideal) with an inverted lid (rounded). Place a stainless steel or heat-safe bowl on tip of brick. Put roses in pot; add enough flowers to reach top of brick. Pour in just enough water to cover roses. Water should be just above the top of brick.

Place lid upside down on pot. Turn on stove and bring water to a rolling boil, then lower heat to a slow, steady simmer. As soon as water begins to boil, toss two or three trays of ice cubes (or a bag of ice) on top of lid.

As water boils, steam rises, hits top of cold lid, and condenses. As water condenses, it flows to center of lid and drops into bowl. Every 20 minutes, quickly lift lid and take out 1or 2 tbsp of rose water. Stop when there is between 1 pint and 1 quart of water that smells and tastes strongly like roses.

If stored in a cool, dark part of pantry, rose water may be kept up to two years, especially if made from distilled water rather than tap water. Rose water can be used in future recipes to sooth or smooth skin or as a cosmetic. If it turns cloudy or does not smell good, discard.

Marshmallow Root Meringue

(Multiple balls)

1 heaping cup unsweetened shredded **coconut**

1 tbsp **Marshmallow Root** powder

2 tbsp honey or maple syrup

4 tbsp **coconut** oil

1 pinch of salt

Chocolate sauce (recipe below)

In a food processor, process shredded **coconut** until gritty. Add remaining ingredients, processing until completely combined.

Scoop balls with ice cream scoop or tablespoon onto parchment paper-lined tray and refrigerate for at least 15 minutes.

Drizzle or dip balls in chocolate sauce. If dipping balls, place in freezer for 10 minutes to harden. If drizzling with chocolate sauce, no need to freeze first.

Chocolate Sauce (double recipe, if also dipping)

2 tbsp **coconut** oil

¼ cup plus 2 tbsp cocoa powder

2 tbsp honey or maple syrup

Melt **coconut** oil in double boiler. Whisk in cocoa powder and honey or maple syrup.

Drizzle (or dip) over meringues, and then refrigerate immediately.

Original Marshmallows

(Approximately 50 marshmallows)

4 tbsp **Marshmallow Root**s (make sure roots are NOT moldy or too woody. Roots provide approximately twice own weight of mucilaginous gel when placed in water.)

2 cups water (or rose water, for aroma)

1¼ cup tragacanth gum (or gum arabic)

1¾ cup sugar

1-2 egg whites, well beaten

Simmer **Marshmallow root**s in water or rose water for 20-30 minutes. Add additional water or rose water if it simmers down. Strain out the roots.

Whip egg whites until stiff.

In a double boiler, heat gum with water/rose water/Marshmallow decoction until dissolved together. Strain with pressure.

Stir in sugar as quickly as possible. When dissolved, add egg whites, stirring constantly, then take off heating element and continue to stir.

Lay out on a flat surface. Let cool and cut into smaller pieces.

Toasted Coconut Marshmallow Ice Cream

(2 servings)

2 bananas, frozen and sliced

⅓ cup full-fat **coconut** milk

3 tbsp brown **rice** protein powder (vanilla flavored)

1 tbsp **Marshmallow Root** powder

1 cup shredded **coconut** flakes, toasted

To make ice cream, blend bananas, **coconut** milk, protein powder, and **Marshmallow Root** powder in a blender or food processor.

Pour into a container with a tight-fitting cover, cover, and put in freezer for 1 hour or until ice cream is firm.

Toast **coconut** in a frying pan over medium heat, stirring constantly until **coconut** turns a golden color.

Remove ice cream from freezer and stir. Scoop out ice cream with an ice cream scoop and form into ice cream balls.

Roll ice cream ball in toasted **coconut** and coat evenly. Repeat until all ice cream has been rolled in **coconut**.

Freeze balls for another 2 hours.

Serve.

Oats, Oat Straw, Oatmeal

This is good old **Oatmeal**. **Oat Straw** is the stalks of **Oats**. Because of the gluten in **Oats** and **Oat Straw**, they are contraindicated in people with celiac disease although gluten-free **Oatmeal** is available.

Oat Straw, Oats (Avenae stramentum)

Type: Minor galactogogue

Medicinal Dose: 100 grams daily

Other Uses: Diuretic and for anxiety and depression

Caution: Do not use if patient has celiac disease.

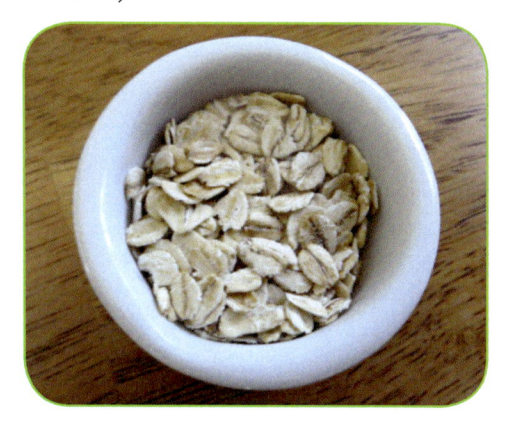

Beverages

Oat and Mango Smoothie

(2 servings)

1 cup boiling water
⅔ cup instant **Oat** flakes
2 mangoes or medium size-canned mango pulp
1 cup milk
½ cup cold water
2 tbsp sugar

Pour boiling water over **Oatmeal**. Stir well, and set aside for 10 minutes.

Cut mangoes in chunks. Placed mango chunks or mango pulp and rest of ingredients in a blender and blend well.

Add soaked **Oatmeal** and blend for 1-2 minutes.

Adjust sweetness level according to taste.

Serve smoothie with ice cubes or chilled.

Breads

Cherry Blueberry Oat Muffins

(12 muffins)

1¼ cups plus 1 tbsp flour
1 cup old fashioned **Oats**
½ cup sugar
½ cup brown sugar
2 tsp baking powder
¼ tsp salt
1 cup buttermilk
¼ cup vegetable oil
1 large egg

1 tsp vanilla extract
½ cup **cherries**, pitted and halved
½ cup blueberries

Preheat oven to 350 degrees.

Line muffin pan with baking cups.

In a large bowl, mix 1¼ cups flour, **Oats**, sugar, brown sugar, baking powder, and salt.

In a medium bowl, mix the buttermilk, oil, egg, and vanilla. Pour into flour mixture and mix until just combined.

Toss **cherries** and blueberries with 1 tbsp flour and fold into batter.

Divide batter evenly into 12 muffin cups.

Bake for 25 minutes.

Pineapple Raisin Oat Bran Muffin

(12 muffins)

Cooking spray, as needed
4 ounces **Oat** bran
⅔ cup dry powder milk (use dry; do NOT add water)
2 eggs
1 tbsp baking powder
1½ tsp baking soda
1 tbsp cinnamon
⅓ cup sugar or honey
1 (20-ounce) can crushed pineapple, undrained
3 ounces raisins
1 **carrot**, shredded (optional)
1 handful almonds, chopped

Preheat oven to 350 degrees.

Spray muffin pan (do NOT use cupcake liners).

Mix rest of ingredients and let sit 20 minutes. Pour batter into 12 muffin cups.

Bake 20-25 minutes (muffins do NOT rise).

Strawberry Jam Oat Squares

(15 squares)

	¾ cup self-rising flour

	2 tsp baking powder

	¾ cup rolled **Oats**

	¼ cup **coconut**

	½ cup sugar

	1 egg

	4 tbsp strawberry jam

	⅓ cup oil

	1 cup sliced strawberries

Preheat oven to 350 degrees.

Sift flour and baking powder into a large mixing bowl. Add **Oats**, **coconut**, and sugar. Mix well.

Beat egg. Add egg, jam, and oil to flour mixture.

Gently stir in strawberries.

Pour into a 13 by 8-inch baking pan and bake for 30 minutes or until an inserted toothpick or knife comes out clean.

Cool and cut into squares.

Breakfasts

Oats Cereal

	(2 servings; Nice family recipe)

	1 cup steel-cut **Oats** (can be presoaked overnight)

	2 cups water or milk

	¼ cup raisins

	¼ cup almonds diced (cut almonds into 2 or 4 parts with knife)

In a saucepan, add water or milk and steel-cut **Oats**. Cover and cook over medium heat, stirring occasionally.

After approximately 10 minutes, reduce heat to simmer and let cook for another 10 minutes.

Remove lid and stir until water evaporates or milk boils, or until desired consistency is reached.

Add raisins and almonds, and serve hot.

Oatmeal Pancakes

(2 servings; Nice family recipe)

½ cup **Oatmeal**

½ cup finely ground almond meal

½ tsp cinnamon, if desired

1 tsp baking powder

⅓ cup ricotta cheese

2 eggs

½ tsp vanilla

½ cup water

Combine **Oatmeal**, almond meal, cinnamon, and baking powder.

In a separate bowl, stir together ricotta cheese, eggs, vanilla, and water. Blend until very smooth.

Add to dry ingredients and stir until well combined.

Batter with be a slightly thicker than regular pancake batter. Can add more water, 1 tbsp at a time, if it appears too thick.

Allow batter to rest, approximately 1 minute; then cook on a griddle or in a large frying pan until golden.

Top with maple syrup or berries and whipped cream.

Oatmeal with Vanilla Soy Milk and Fresh Berries

(2 servings; Nice family recipe)

1 cup rolled **Oats**

1¼ cups boiling water

¼ cup vanilla soy milk (or any other type of vanilla milk – **coconut**, almond, etc.)

¼ tsp vanilla extract

1 tbsp brown sugar or 2 packages sugar substitute

¼ tsp cinnamon

¼ cup blueberries

¼ cup **Red Raspberries**

In a nonstick saucepan, add **Oats** and cook over medium heat, approximately 2 minutes to toast. Stir often.

Add boiling water and reduce heat to a simmer. Simmer on low for 5 minutes or until most of liquid is absorbed, stirring occasionally.

Stir in soy milk and vanilla, and continue to simmer, approximately 3 minutes, until desired consistency. Add more soy milk, if desired.

Stir in brown sugar or sugar substitute and cinnamon.

Spoon into serving bowl and top with blueberries and **Red Raspberries**.

Soups

Oatmeal Chicken Soup

(6 servings)

1 (1-pound) chicken, cut up

8 cups water

1 medium onion, sliced

1 **Garlic** clove, minced

1 tbsp chili powder

3 green cardamoms

2 chicken bouillon cubes

1 tsp salt

3 tbsp tomato paste

1½ cups **Oats**

1-2 tbsp vegetable oil

1 tsp **cumin** seeds

Combine first 8 ingredients in a large pan. Simmer for 30 minutes or until chicken is tender.

Remove chicken and let cool. When cool, debone and shred.

Strain broth into a large pot. Add shredded chicken and tomato paste. Simmer for 5 minutes.

Add **Oats** and simmer for 10 minutes. Stir frequently to keep **oatmeal** from sticking to bottom of pot.

Heat oil in a small skillet. Toast **cumin** seeds in hot oil until fragrant. Pour over hot soup.

Serve.

Entrees

Oat Battered Fried Chicken with Garlic Mayonnaise

(4 servings)

1 small whole chicken, washed and cut into pieces

Your favorite batter

1 cup **Oats**

1 cup corn flakes

2 eggs, beaten

Vegetable oil

1 **Garlic** clove, chopped

½ cup mayonnaise

Dry chicken with cloth or paper towel.

Crush corn flakes and **oats** together in a dish large enough to coat chicken pieces.

In another dish large enough to dip chicken pieces, beat eggs.

Dip dried chicken pieces in beaten egg, then coat with Oat cornflake mixture.

Heat oil in skillet. Fry battered chicken pieces until golden brown.

In a small skillet, heat oil. Add **Garlic** and sauté until color changes slightly. Add to mayonnaise and mix well.

Serve fried chicken with **garlic** mayonnaise.

Oat Crusted Chicken with Dill

(2 servings)

1½ tbsp milk
1 tsp mustard
¼ cup rolled **Oats**
2 tbsp fresh **Dill**, chopped (divided)
Salt, to taste (divided)
Ground black pepper, to taste (divided)
4 chicken drumsticks, skinned
¼ cup ricotta cheese
1 tbsp Dijon mustard
1 tbsp sour cream

Preheat oven to 400 degrees.

In a small bowl, mix together milk and mustard.

On a plate, mix **Oats**, salt, and pepper with half of the chopped **Dill**.

Brush chicken with milk mustard mixture and coat evenly with **Oat** mixture.

Place chicken on a baking sheet. Bake approximately 40 minutes, or until done.

Mix together ricotta cheese, Dijon mustard, and rest of chopped **Dill** in a bowl to make sauce. Season with salt and pepper.

Serve chicken with ricotta sauce.

Turkey Meatloaf

(4 servings)

1 pound ground turkey
1 egg
1 tbsp seasoning blend, to taste
½ tsp powdered **Ginger**
1 cup quick **Oats**
⅓ cup golden breadcrumbs (adjust for consistency)
Cooking spray, as needed

Preheat oven to 325 degrees.

Spray a loaf pan lightly with cooking spray.

In a bowl, combine turkey, egg, seasoning blend, and **Ginger**. Mix well.

Add **Oats** and mix until well incorporated (no dry spots).

Add breadcrumbs gradually until mixture will hold in a loose ball.

Place in loaf pan and bake for 60 minutes, or until done.

Cool slowly, and when comfortable to touch, serve.

Note: To blend flavors even more, cover tightly with plastic wrap or tight sealing lid and refrigerate overnight.

Zucchini Quiche

(8 servings)

Crust

- 2 cups flour
- 2 tbsp **Oats**
- 3 tbsp butter
- 2 tbsp Crisco
- 4 tbsp cold water (plus more, if needed, to bind dough)

Filling

- 1 large zucchini, shredded
- 1 small red onion, sliced thin
- 2 **Garlic** cloves, peeled and chopped
- ½ cup grated Parmesan cheese (divided)
- 2 dashes salt
- 2 dashes ground black pepper
- 4 ounces cheddar cheese, shredded
- 5 eggs, beaten
- Splash of milk

Preheat oven to 350 degrees.

To make crust, place flour in a large bowl along with **Oats**. Add butter and

Crisco and work with fingers to form small pieces.

Add water to begin to bind dough. Add water as needed until dough is formed. Form into a ball.

Dust a clean flat surface with flour and roll out dough to fit a 9-inch pie plate.

Bake crust for 10-12 minutes. Let cool.

To make filling, combine zucchini, onion, **Garlic**, ¼ cup Parmesan cheese, salt, pepper, and cheddar cheese in a large bowl.

In a separate bowl, beat eggs and milk.

Pour egg mixture into zucchini mixture and combine.

Pour zucchini mixture into piecrust and top with rest of Parmesan cheese.

Bake 35-40 minutes or until firm in middle.

Desserts

Apple Custard Pie

(8 servings)

Crust

1 cup **Oats**

½ cup all-purpose flour

¼ tsp cinnamon

¼ cup brown sugar

4 tbsp butter, softened

Filling

2 eggs

¼ cup sugar

½ tsp vanilla extract

¾ cup milk

3 apples, peeled and cut into wedges

¼ tsp cinnamon

Topping

 1 tbsp flour

 1 tbsp brown sugar

 1 tbsp sugar

 1 tsp cinnamon

Preheat oven to 350 degrees.

To make crust, process **Oats**, flour, cinnamon, and brown sugar in a food processor until **Oats** are ground.

Pour Oat mixture into a large bowl, add butter, and mix until dough is crumbly.

Pour into a buttered pie pan. Press dough evenly into bottom and sides to form crust.

Bake 15 minutes or until crust is light golden brown. Remove from oven and let cool.

To make filling, beat together eggs, sugar, and vanilla. Add milk and beat until smooth.

Arrange apple wedges on bottom of crust. Sprinkle with cinnamon. Pour egg mixture over apples.

To make topping, combine flour, brown sugar, sugar, and cinnamon. Sprinkle on top of pie.

Return to oven and bake for 30-40 minutes, or until filling is set.

Black Cherry Crumble

 (8-10 servings)

 ½ cup **cherry** cordial (Cherry Kijafa is a fine option or use Polish brand, 'Wisniowka' (vish-NOV-kuh)

 1 can black **cherries** (reserve juice)

 ½ cup almond slices

 ½ cup sugar

 ¼ cup plus 3 tbsp tapioca flour or all purpose flour

 6 cups pitted fresh black (Bing) **cherries** (or frozen, thawed)

 ½ cup dark brown sugar, packed

1 cup quick-cooking **Oats**

2 tbsp plus ¼ cup sweet butter, softened

½ tsp ground cinnamon

Preheat the oven to 350 degrees. Grease a 9 x 13 x 2-inch ovenproof dish with 2 tbsp butter.

Bring **cherry** cordial and reserved **cherry** juice to a boil. Reduce liquid to approximately ¼ to ½ cup. Remove from heat and set aside.

Sauté almond slices over medium heat until they are golden brown. Set aside.

Whisk together white sugar and 3 tbsp tapioca or all-purpose flour in a large bowl. Add canned **cherries**, fresh **cherries**, and **cherry** cordial reduction.

Pour **cherry** mixture into buttered dish.

Combine brown sugar, ¼ cup tapioca or all-purpose flour, and **Oats** in a bowl. Cut in ¼ cup softened butter to make a crumble. Add toasted almonds. Pour evenly over **cherries**.

Sprinkle ground cinnamon evenly over topping.

Bake approximately 35 minutes, until topping is brown.

Let rest for at least 15 minutes.

Serve with a scoop of vanilla ice cream.

Chocolate Banana Oat Cake

(8 servings)

1 egg

2½ tbsp vegetable oil

½ cup sugar

3 overripe bananas (divided)

¾ cup flour, sifted

¼ cup rolled **Oats** (divided)

¼ cup dark chocolate, grated

1 tsp cinnamon

½ tsp baking powder

½ tsp baking soda

Preheat oven to 350 degrees.

Whisk egg, oil, and sugar.

Mash 2 bananas. Add to egg mixture and mix well.

Add flour, ⅛ cup **oats**, chocolate, cinnamon, baking powder, and baking soda and mix well.

Pour into a greased 8-inch round cake pan. Top with sliced banana and rest of **Oats**.

Bake approximately 30-40 minutes, until an inserted toothpick comes out clean.

Chocolate Banana Peanut Butter Oatmeal Cookies

(Approximately 32 cookies)

¼ cup butter, softened

½ cup brown sugar, packed

⅓ cup granulated sugar

¼ cup peanut butter, softened

2 large eggs

2 medium, overripe bananas

1 tbsp vanilla extract

1½ cups flour

½ cup cocoa powder

½ tsp baking soda

½ tsp salt

1 cup **Oats**

1 cup peanuts, chopped

2 dried apricots, chopped

In a large bowl, cream together butter, brown sugar, sugar, and peanut butter. Add eggs, bananas, and vanilla extract. Beat until well combined. Set aside.

In a medium bowl, sift together flour, cocoa power, baking soda, and salt. Gradually add to butter mixture.

Add **Oats** and mix well.

Refrigerate for at least 30 minutes.

When ready to bake, preheat oven to 350 degrees.

Line two large baking sheets with parchment paper.

Form 16 rounded mounds of dough on each cookie sheet. Arrange approximately 2 inches apart. Top each cookie with a sprinkle of peanuts and apricots if desired. Press peanuts/apricots lightly into dough.

Bake one tray at a time for approximately 15 minutes. Once out of oven, leave cookies on sheet for 5 more minutes before transferring to a wire rack.

Let cool at room temperature before eating or storing.

Cookies may be stored at room temperature for approximately one week or frozen for up to three months.

Crockpot Apple Crisp

(8 servings)

10 large apples, cut in wedges

½ cup white sugar

1⅔ cup brown sugar (divided)

1 tbsp apple pie spice

⅔ cup old fashion **Oats**

¼ cup flour

½ tsp cinnamon

2 tsp vanilla

4 tbsp butter, softened

In a large bowl, combine white sugar, 1 cup brown sugar, and apple pie spice. Add apple wedges and coat with sugar. Put mixture into Crockpot.

In a bowl, combine **Oats**, ⅔ cup brown sugar, flour, cinnamon, and vanilla. Add butter.

Sprinkle over top of apple mixture.

Turn Crockpot on Low for 4 hours or High for 2 hours. Cook until apples are soft. Juice will thicken as crumble cools.

Quinoa

Quinoa seeds are high in protein and are considered a complete vegetarian diet. It is a grain that has been used by ethnic societies to increase milk production during lactation. **Quinoa** is gluten free.

Quinoa (Chenopodium quinoa)

Type: Minor galactogogue

Medicinal Dose: 45 grams daily

Other Uses: For constipation, diabetes, hypertension, and high cholesterol; as an antioxidant

Caution: Risks are minimal provided leaves are not eaten in excess (contain oxalic acid).

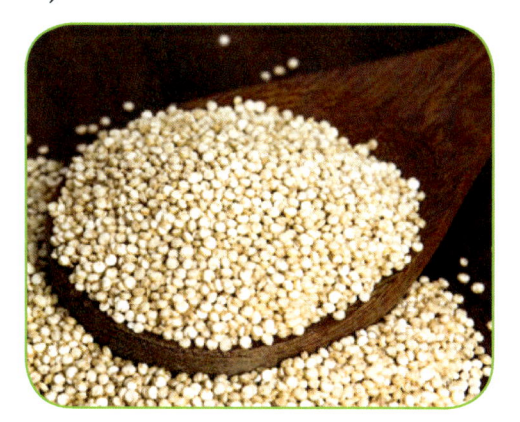

Salads

Hijiki Salad

(4 servings)

½ cup dry hijiki (Japanese **seaweed**)

1 cup cherry tomatoes, halved

1 cup corn, cooked

1 cup **peas**, cooked

1 small red onion, sliced in thin half moons

½ cup hard tofu, diced

1 tbsp extra-virgin olive oil

¼ tsp sesame oil

3 tbsp lemon juice

1 tsp prepared mustard

Ground black pepper, to taste

¼ cup **Quinoa**

½ cup **chicken stock** or water

Place **Quinoa** in mesh strainer and rinse under cold water.

Place **chicken stock** or water in a saucepan and bring to a boil.

Add **Quinoa**, lower heat, and let simmer for 15 minutes or until liquid is absorbed. Fluff with fork. Set aside.

Rinse hijiki. Drain and cover with fresh water. Let soak for 15 minutes. Drain and slice.

In a large salad bowl, combine tomatoes, corn, **peas**, onion, tofu, and hijiki.

In a small bowl, whisk olive oil, sesame oil, lemon juice, and mustard until emulsified.

Add dressing to salad and toss.

Sprinkle **Quinoa** on salad.

Quinoa and Dill Salad

(4 servings)

3 cups water

1½ cups **Quinoa**

1 small red onion, diced into ¼ inch pieces

2 tbsp fresh **Dill**, finely snipped, or 4 tsp dried **Dill**

½ cup extra virgin olive oil

¼ cup red wine vinegar

1 lemon, juiced

1½ tsp salt

¾ tsp freshly ground black pepper

4 Romaine **lettuce** leaves

1 avocado, seeded and sliced

1 cracked black pepper for garnish (optional)

Bring water to boil in large saucepan.

Add **Quinoa**, stir once, and return to boil. Cook, uncovered, over moderate heat for 10 minutes.

Strain and rinse well with cool water. Shake the sieve well to remove all moisture.

When dry, transfer **Quinoa** to large bowl. Add red onion and **Dill**, and mix well.

In a small bowl, whisk together olive oil, red wine vinegar, lemon juice, salt, and ground black pepper. Pour over **Quinoa** mixture and toss well to coat.

Serve on **lettuce** lined plates, topped with avocado and cracked black pepper.

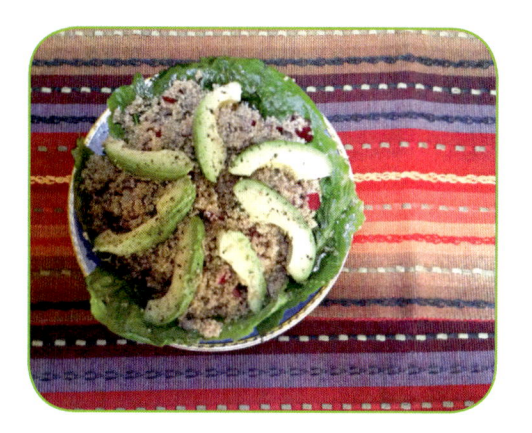

Quinoa, Chickpea, and Kale Salad

(4 servings)

1 cup **Quinoa**

2 cups **chicken stock**/broth or water

3 tbsp plus ⅓ cup olive oil, divided

1 bunch kale leaves, torn

1 shallot, finely chopped

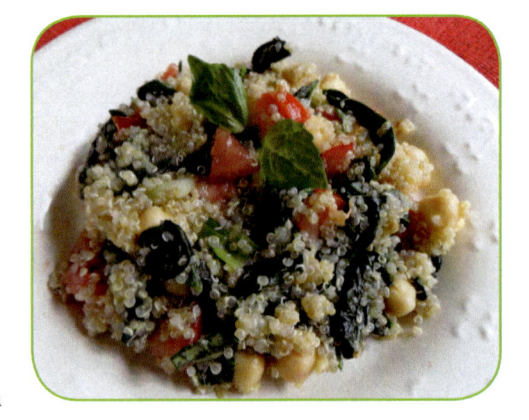

1 (14½ ounce) can **chickpeas** (garbanzo beans), drained and rinsed

1 medium tomato, chopped and diced

5-6 fresh **basil** leaves, chopped

1 pinch salt, to taste

1 pinch tsp ground black pepper, to taste

zest of ½ lemon (colored portion of peel)

1 lemon, juiced

Place **Quinoa** in mesh strainer and rinse under cold water.

In a saucepan, bring **chicken stock**/broth or water to a boil.

Add **Quinoa**, cover, and simmer for 15 minutes or until liquid is absorbed. Remove from heat and fluff with fork.

In a large skillet, heat 3 tbsp olive oil.

Add kale and shallots and cook until slightly wilted.

Transfer cooked kale and shallots to a large mixing bowl.

Add **Quinoa**, **chickpeas** (garbanzo beans), tomatoes, **basil**, salt, and pepper. Toss until well combined.

In a small bowl, whisk lemon zest, lemon juice, and ⅓ cup olive oil.

Pour dressing over **Quinoa** mixture and toss to coat.

Note: For a robust nutty flavor, toast **Quinoa** in a dry skillet, stirring often, until lightly browned, before adding cooking liquid.

Sweet Potato Quinoa Cakes on Salad Greens

(5 servings)

2 medium baked **sweet potatoes** (skins discarded)

2 cups cooked **quinoa**

2 scallions, chopped

2 **garlic** cloves, minced

½ tsp sea salt

½ tsp crushed red pepper

½ tsp black pepper

1 tsp **cumin**

¼ cup olive oil

5 servings salad greens, washed

Favorite salad dressing

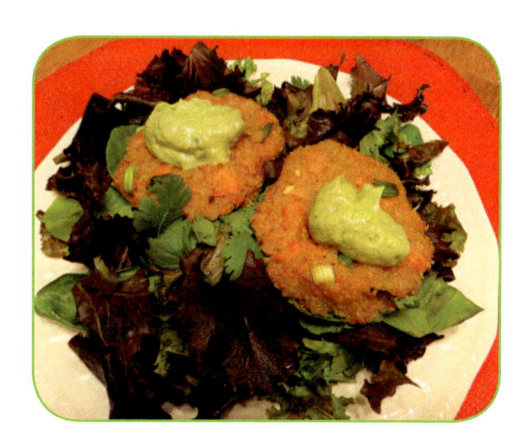

Preheat oven to 350 degrees.

In a large bowl, mash **sweet potatoes**. Stir in **quinoa**, scallions, **garlic**, salt, red pepper, black pepper, and **cumin**, stirring to thoroughly combine ingredients.

Shape **quinoa** mixture into palm-sized patties and place on non-stick baking sheet.

Brush tops with olive oil.

Bake for 10-15 minutes or until golden brown.

Lightly dress salad greens with favorite salad dressing. Divide salad greens on 5 plates.

Place 2 patties on top of salad greens on each plate. Place a dollop of the avocado dressing (below) on top of each patty.

Serve.

Avocado Dressing

(6 servings)

1 avocado, peel and pit removed

1 tbsp sesame tahini

1 tbsp olive oil

10 cilantro leaves

Juice of 1 lime

¼ tsp crushed red pepper

Place all ingredients in blender and pulse until smooth (about 1-2 minutes).

If mixture is too thick, add small amounts of water until desired consistency is reached.

Refrigerate until ready to use.

Soups

Quinoa Hearty Galactogogue Vegetable Soup

(6 servings)

½ cup **Quinoa**

1 cup **chicken stock/**broth or water, plus 2 cups **chicken stock/**broth plus 2 cups water

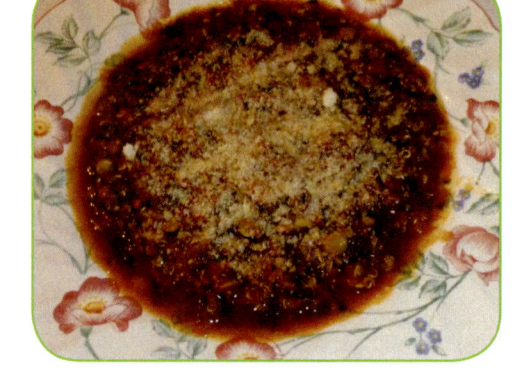

1 (14½ ounce) can stewed tomatoes, Italian seasoned, drained and liquid reserved

1 cup vegetable bouillon from cube

⅓ cup brown **lentils**, rinsed

2 tbsp split **peas**, rinsed

½ tsp extra virgin olive oil

1 tsp ground black pepper

1 bay leaf, whole

1 **Fennel** stock with frond, whole

1 leafy celery (approximately 3 inch piece), whole

1 onion

2 **Garlic** cloves

1 **carrot**

1 Italian turkey sausage link

2 cups fresh **spinach**, minced

2 tbsp fresh **Coriander** leaves (cilantro)

½ tsp **basil**

2 tsp **Anise**

¼ tsp orange zest (colored potion of peel)

1 tsp salt, to taste

¼ cup Parmesan cheese, grated

Place **Quinoa** in mesh strainer and rinse under cold water.

In a saucepan, bring 1 cup **chicken stock**/broth or water to a boil.

Add **Quinoa**, cover, and simmer for 15 minutes or until liquid is absorbed. Remove from heat and fluff with fork.

In a soup pot, combine liquid from stewed tomatoes, 2 cups **chicken stock**/broth, and 1 cup vegetable bouillon.

Add **lentils**, **peas**, olive oil, pepper, bay leaf, **Fennel**, and celery. Bring to a boil. Reduce heat and simmer until **lentils** are tender, approximately 20 to 25 minutes.

In a food processor, finely chop onion, **Garlic**, and **carrot**.

In large skillet, on medium heat, cook drained tomatoes, onion, **Garlic**, and carrot until slightly caramelized and aromatic.

Add Italian turkey sausage link. Brown and crumble meat.

From soup, remove **Fennel** frond, celery, and bay leaf. Add sausage mixture and 2 cups water. Simmer approximately 15 to 25 minutes.

Add cooked **Quinoa**, **spinach**, **Coriander** leaves (cilantro), **basil**, **Anise**, and orange zest. Simmer until **spinach** is just wilted.

Serve in bowl, topped with Parmesan cheese.

Note: For a robust nutty flavor, toast **Quinoa** in dry skillet, stirring often, approximately 5 minutes, before adding cooking liquid.

Entrees

Baked Quinoa Casserole with Potatoes and Cheese

(4-6 servings)

1 cup **Quinoa**

2 cups **chicken stock**/broth or water

1 pound red potatoes, unpeeled, diced into small pieces

2 tbsp extra virgin olive oil

2 leeks white part, thinly sliced

2 **Garlic** cloves, peeled and diced

1 green bell pepper, diced into small pieces

4 large eggs

¾ cup low fat milk

½ tsp salt, to taste

½ tsp pepper, to taste

1½ cups smoked cheddar cheese, grated

Preheat oven to 350 degrees. Oil 2-quart casserole baking dish.

Place **Quinoa** in mesh strainer and rinse under cold water.

In a saucepan, add **chicken stock**/broth or water and bring to a boil. Add **Quinoa**, cover, and simmer for 15 minutes or until liquid is absorbed. Remove from heat and fluff with fork.

Place diced potatoes in a saucepan, cover with water. Bring to a boil, reduce to a simmer, and cook until tender. Drain and set aside.

In a sauté pan over medium heat, heat olive oil and add leeks. Sauté, stirring until tender, approximately 5 minutes.

Add **Garlic** and continue to cook, stirring for 1 minute.

Add peppers and cook, covered, for 5 to 10 minutes, until peppers are tender, yet crisp. Remove from heat.

In a mixing bowl, beat eggs and low fat milk.

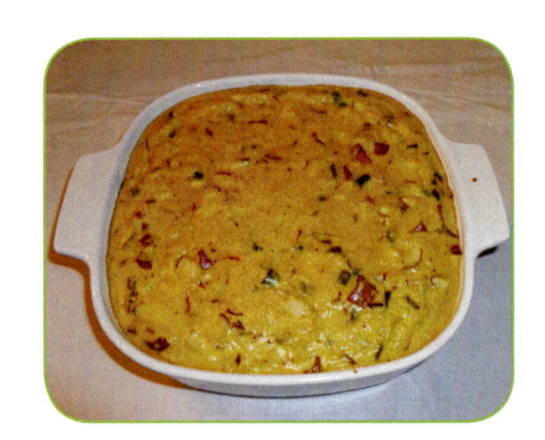

Stir in **Quinoa**, cheese, red potatoes, leek/pepper mixture, salt, and pepper.

Pour into greased baking dish. Bake covered for 45 minutes.

Remove cover and bake approximately 15 minutes or until top is golden.

Let mixture rest approximately 5 minutes before serving.

Note: For a robust nutty flavor, toast **Quinoa** in dry skillet, stirring often, approximately 5 minutes, before adding cooking liquid.

Quinoa, Lima Bean, and Corn Casserole

(4 servings)

¾ cup **Quinoa**

1½ cups **chicken stock**/broth or water

1 box (9 ounces) frozen baby lima beans, cooked according to package directions

1 box (10 ounces) frozen corn, cooked according to package directions

1 tbsp butter

1 tsp paprika

2 medium plum (Roma) tomatoes, seeded and chopped

½ tsp salt

¼ tsp ground black pepper

2 thinly sliced green onions, if desired

Place **Quinoa** in mesh strainer and rinse under cold water.

In a saucepan, bring **chicken stock**/broth or water to a boil. Add **Quinoa**, cover, and simmer for 15 minutes or until liquid is absorbed. Remove from heat and fluff with fork.

In a skillet, add lima beans, corn, butter, paprika, **Quinoa**, tomato, salt, and pepper. Mix well. Cook over medium heat, stirring frequently, until mixture is thoroughly heated.

To serve, garnish with green onions if desired.

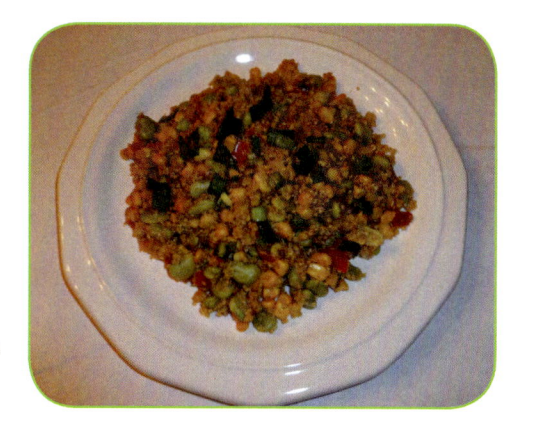

Note: For a robust nutty flavor, toast **Quinoa** in dry skillet, stirring often, approximately 5 minutes, before adding cooking liquid.

Quinoa Patties with Mustard Dill Sauce

(8 servings)

4 tbsp prepared dark mustard, highly seasoned

1 tsp dry mustard powder

3 tbsp sugar

2 tbsp white vinegar

$1/3$ cup vegetable oil

3 tbsp fresh **Dill**, chopped, or 6 tsp dried **Dill**, plus portion for garnish

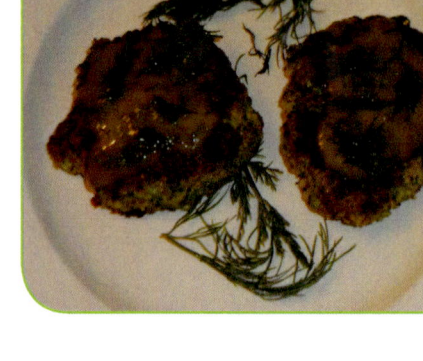

½ cup **Quinoa**

1 cup **chicken stock**/broth or water

2 cups broccoli, steamed until softened, and chopped into small pieces

2 eggs

½ cup seasoned Italian bread crumbs

¼ cup Parmesan cheese, grated

2 tbsp olive oil, plus more for frying

1 pinch salt, to taste

1 pinch ground black pepper, to taste

In a small bowl, combine prepared mustard, dry mustard, sugar, white vinegar, vegetable oil, and **Dill**. Refrigerate to blend flavors until ready to use.

Place **Quinoa** in mesh strainer and rinse under cold water.

In a saucepan, bring **chicken stock**/broth or water to a boil. Add **Quinoa**, cover, and simmer for 15 minutes or until liquid is absorbed. Remove from heat and fluff with fork.

Steam broccoli in a steamer or in the microwave until soft.

In a mixing bowl, beat eggs, olive oil, salt, and pepper. Add broccoli, **Quinoa**, bread crumbs, and Parmesan cheese, and mix well. Form into 8 patties.

In an nonstick skillet with a little oil, sauté patties until browned.

Serve with mustard **Dill** sauce, with additional **Dill** sprinkled on top.

Note: For a robust nutty flavor, toast **Quinoa** in dry skillet, stirring often, approximately 5 minutes, before adding cooking liquid.

Sides

Quinoa with Carrots, and Peas

(4 servings)

2 tsp olive oil or canola oil

1 **Garlic** clove, chopped

1 cup **Quinoa**

2 cups **chicken stock**/broth or water

1 tbsp fresh **Dill** or 2 tsp dried **Dill**

1 tsp ground black pepper

1 large **carrot**, chopped

1cup **peas**

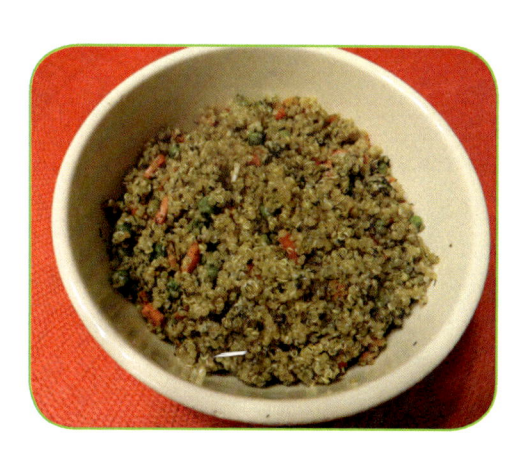

Heat oil in sauce pan over medium heat. Add **Garlic** and cook until translucent.

Lower heat, stir in **Quinoa** and toast, stirring constantly, for no more than 2 minutes.

Stir in **chicken stock**/broth or water, **Dill**, and black pepper, and bring to a boil. Cover, reduce heat to low, and simmer for 5 minutes.

Stir in **carrots** and **peas**.

Cover and simmer until all water is absorbed, approximately 10 minutes.

Serve as side dish or with salad.

Red Clover

The use of the fermented form of **Red Clover** may result in increased estrogenic properties.

Red Clover (Trifolium pretense)

Type: Minor galactogogue

Medicinal Dose: 40 mg to 80 mg daily as tincture or tea

Other Uses: For estrogenic properties and as expectorant

Caution: Do not exceed recommended dosage; avoid fermented **Red Clover**; patients taking anticoagulants and/or aspirin should not use (contains coumarin, a blood thinner).

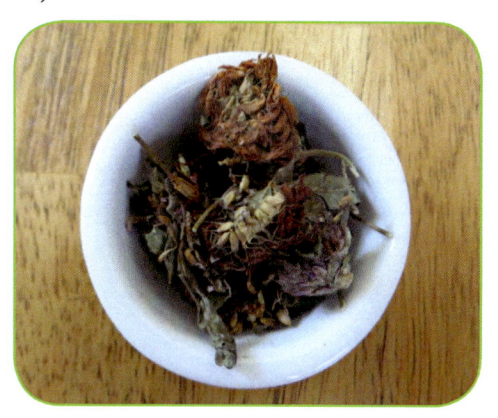

Beverages

Herb Tea

(1 serving; herbal remedy)

2 parts bergamot (fruit the size of an orange with a yellow color similar to a lemon)
1 part **lemon balm** (check on-line)
1 part apple mint (perennial herb)
1 large pinch Roman chamomile flowers
1 large pinch **Red Clover** flowers

Blend herbs together.
Use 1 tsp per cup of boiling water (can be chilled and served as iced tea).

Red Clover Lemonade

(4 servings; herbal remedy)

3 cups **Red Clover** blooms
4 cups water
1¼ cups lemon juice
4 tbsp honey

Boil **Red Clover** blooms and water for 5-7 minutes.
Strain blooms from water.
Add lemon juice and honey. Stir and chill for 1-2 hours.
To serve, pour over ice.

Red Clover Tea

(1 serving; herbal remedy)

1 tsp dried **Red Clover** flowers
1 cup boiling water
1 tsp daisy petals

Honey, to taste

1 cinnamon stick, for garnish

Mix dried **Red Clover** flowers with hot water.

Add daisy petals and honey. Steep for 15 minutes.

Strain flowers and petals.

Garnish with cinnamon stick.

Breads

Red Clover Corn Bread

(8 servings)

1 cup cornmeal

1 cup unbleached flour

2 tsp baking powder

½ tsp baking soda

½ tsp coarse salt

1 egg

1 cup yogurt

3 tbsp honey

3 tbsp extra-virgin olive oil

1 cup fresh **Red Clover** blossoms, finely chopped

Preheat oven to 350 degrees.

Butter an 8-inch square baking pan.

In a large bowl, combine cornmeal, flour, baking powder, baking soda, and salt in a mixing bowl.

In a small bowl, beat egg lightly and add yogurt, honey, and olive oil.

Add egg mixture to dry ingredients, stirring just until thoroughly mixed. (If mixture is not moist enough to mix, add a little milk.)

Fold in **Red Clover** blossoms.

Spread mixture into baking pan.

Bake for 20 minutes or until top is golden and center is firm to touch.

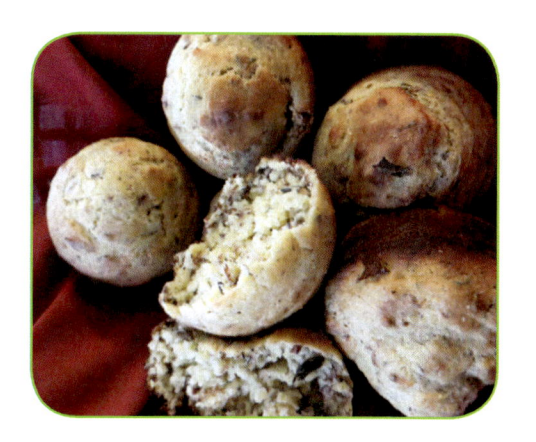

Condiments

Red Clover Jelly 1

(2 pints or 4 half pint jars)

Infusion

    4 cups boiling water

    4 cups **Red Clover** flower heads (some parts of greens are acceptable)

Place **Red Clover** in a glass or stainless steel container, cover with boiling water, and steep overnight.

Strain out flowers and squeeze out excess water, reserving liquid for jelly.

Jelly

    4 cups **Red Clover** infusion (add water to replace what was lost in straining)

    8 tbsp lemon juice

    2 packages powdered pectin

    8 cups sugar

Add lemon juice to infusion, stir in pectin, and bring to a boil, stirring frequently.

Add sugar all at once and bring to a rolling boil. Boil for 1 minute, skim, and pour into jelly jars.

Process like any other jelly in a hot water bath.

Red Clover Jelly 2

(2 pints or 4 half pint jars)

Infusion

    5 cups apple juice or white wine

    2 cups **Red Clover** flower heads (some parts of greens are acceptable)

Place **Red Clover** in a glass or stainless steel container.

Bring juice or wine to a boil and pour over **Red Clover**.

Cover and let sit until cool (overnight is acceptable).

Strain out flowers and squeeze out excess water, reserving liquid for jelly.

Jelly

> 4 cups **Red Clover** infusion (add water to replace what was lost in straining)
>
> 8 cups sugar
>
> ½ cup lemon juice
>
> 6 ounces liquid pectin

Combine infusion, sugar, and lemon juice.

Bring to a boil over high heat. As soon as sugar has dissolved, stir in pectin.

Return to a rolling boil for 1 minute.

Remove from heat, skim foam, and pour into jelly jars.

Process like any other jelly in a hot water bath.

Salads

Red Clover Spinach Salad

> (4 servings)
>
> 2 cups baby **spinach**
>
> ½-1 cup grape tomatoes
>
> ½ cup strawberries, chopped
>
> ¼ cup blueberries
>
> ¼ cup kiwi or mandarin oranges, chopped
>
> ½ cup **Red Clover** sprouts
>
> 1 small apple, chopped,
>
> ¼ cup almond slivers
>
> 3 tbsp **Red Raspberry** vinaigrette dressing (see Condiments under **Red Raspberry** for recipe)
>
> ¼ cup feta cheese or bleu (or blue) cheese
>
> ¼ cup chia seeds

Combine **spinach**, tomatoes, strawberries, blueberries, kiwi or mandarin oranges, **Red Clover** sprouts, apple, and almond slivers in a large bowl.

Toss with **Red Raspberry** vinaigrette dressing.

Top with feta or bleu cheese and chia seeds.

Entrees

Asian Noodles

(4 servings; Korean ancestors' remedy)

8 ounce Udon (Japanese wheat noodles) noodles or spaghetti

1 tbsp cornstarch

3 tbsp cool water

⅓ cup tamari or soy sauce

1 tbsp dark roasted sesame oil

1 tbsp mirin or seasoned **rice** vinegar

2 tsp fresh **Ginger** root, chopped

2 tsp **Garlic** cloves, chopped

1 tsp sugar

½ tsp crushed red pepper flakes

1 (10½ ounce) package extra-hard tofu, cut into pieces ½ inch thick, long, and wide

4 ounces **mung**, **lentil**, or adzuki sprouts (or combination)

4 ounces **Red Clover** sprouts

Cook noodles according to package directions. Drain. Keep warm.

In medium bowl, combine cornstarch and water, mixing until smooth. Stir in tamari or soy sauce, sesame oil, mirin or seasoned **rice** vinegar, **Ginger**, **Garlic**, sugar, and pepper flakes; mix well.

Heat a large nonstick skillet over medium-high heat.

Stir-fry tofu in tamari or soy sauce mix until tofu is warm and sauce thickens, approximately 2-3 minutes.

Add in **mung**, **lentils**, or adzuki sprouts (or combination) and **Red Clover** sprouts; stir-fry just until sprouts are heated through, approximately 1 minute.

Place noodles in serving bowl. Top with tofu mixture and toss to mix.

Red Clover Burritos

(8 servings)

- 4 ounces soft cream cheese
- 2 tbsp plain yogurt or low-fat sour cream
- 1½ tbsp fresh lemon juice
- ¾ tsp dry **Dill** weed
- ½ tsp Dijon mustard
- 8 flour tortillas (7-inch diameter)
- 1 small cucumber, very thinly sliced
- 2 cups **Red Clover** sprouts
- ¾ pound tiny cooked shrimp or smoked salmon
- ¾ cup frozen **peas**, thawed
- 1 approximately 4-ounce can jar ripe olives, sliced

In a small bowl, combine cream cheese, yogurt or sour cream, lemon juice, **Dill**, and mustard.

Lay tortillas flat on a work surface.

Spread 1 tbsp of cream cheese mixture over each tortilla, covering completely.

Proportionately layer cucumber and **Red Clover** sprouts over cheese, leaving about 1 inch clear along bottom and right side.

Lay shrimp or smoked salmon, **peas**, and olives side by side down center of tortilla to within 1 inch of bottom.

Fold left side over center and then, right side over to create a cone.

Red Raspberry

Red Raspberry may decrease milk supply after more than two weeks of use due to its astringent properties. Both **Red Raspberry** fruit and leaves are used.

Red Raspberry (Rubi idaei folium)

Type: Minor galactogogue

Medicinal Dose: 2.7 grams as three (3) 300 mg capsules 3 times a day or daily as tincture or tea

Other Uses: Nutritive

Caution: Red Raspberry rarely may cause loose stools and/or nausea; may decrease milk supply if used for greater than two weeks.

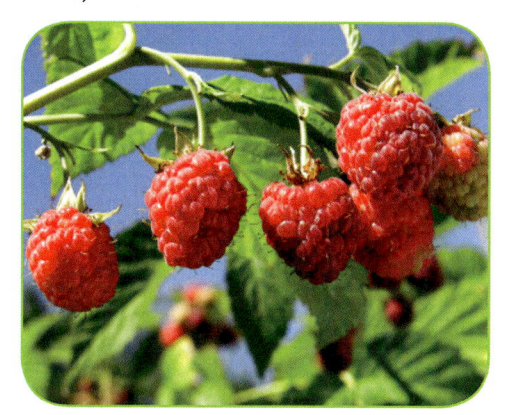

Beverages

Red Raspberry Tea

(10 servings; herbal remedy)

1 gallon boiling water
10 **Red Raspberry** tea bags
3 tbsp fructose
Honey, to taste

Pour hot boiling water over tea bags. Let steep 5-10 minutes.
Add in fructose and fold in honey.

Condiments

Red Raspberry Honey Vinegar

(Approximately 8 half pint jars)

4 cups **Red Raspberries**
4 cups white wine vinegar (divided)
¼ cup sugar
¼ cup honey

Combine **Red Raspberries** and 1 cup white wine vinegar in a glass bowl. Lightly crush **Red Raspberries**.

Stir in remaining white wine vinegar, sugar, and honey.

Cover bowl with waxed paper or plastic wrap and secure. Let vinegar steep in a cold, dark place for 4 weeks, stirring every 2-3 days.

Prepare canning jars and closures according to manufacturer's instructions.

Strain vinegar through several layers of damp cheesecloth. Heat vinegar to a simmer (do NOT boil).

Carefully ladle warm vinegar into warm jars, leaving ¼-inch headspace. Wipe jar rim clean. Place lid on jar with sealing compound next to glass. Screw band down firmly just until a point of resistance is met that is fingertip tight.

Process 10 minutes in a boiling-water canner (at elevations higher than 1,000 feet, boil 2 additional minutes for each additional 1,000 feet elevation).

May add ¼ cup washed, fresh **Red Raspberries** to each jar before filling with flavored vinegar.

Process according to canning instructions.

Red Raspberry Jam

(Approximately 8 half pint jars)

5 cups **Red Raspberries**, crushed

½ tsp butter

1 box fruit pectin

7 cups sugar

Sterilize jars and lids.

Crush **Red Raspberries**; press pulp through sieve to remove seeds if desired.

Combine **Red Raspberries**, butter, and fruit pectin in large pot.

Bring to a full rolling boil, stirring constantly. Add sugar.

Return to full rolling boil and boil 1 minute, stirring constantly. Remove from heat. Skim off any foam.

Fill jars quickly to ⅛ inch of tops. Wipe jar rims. Cover quickly with flat lids. Screw bands tightly.

Invert jars for 5 minutes; then turn upright. After 60 minutes, check seals.

Red Raspberry Vinaigrette Dressing

¼ cup **Red Raspberry** vinegar

½ cup **Red Raspberries**, fresh or frozen, pureed

1 **Garlic** clove, minced

1 tsp honey

3 tbsp water

¼ cup extra-virgin olive oil

Coarse salt, to taste

Fresh ground black pepper, to taste

In a bowl, mix **Red Raspberry** vinegar with **Red Raspberries**.

Add **Garlic** and honey.

Whisk in water and oil until mixture is smooth.

Season with salt and pepper to taste.

Salads

Salad with Red Raspberry Vinaigrette Dressing

(1 serving)

1 portion greens (assorted hearts of romaine **lettuce**, bib **lettuce**, iceberg **lettuce**, and/or **spinach**)

1 portion fresh cleaned **carrots**, celery, peppers, **beets**, **chickpeas** (garbanzo beans), tomatoes, broccoli, cucumbers, and/or beans

Red Raspberry vinaigrette dressing (recipe above)

1 tbsp **almonds**, walnuts, or hazelnuts, for topping

1 tbsp feta cheese

Place greens on a plate.

Top with vegetables.

Drizzle dressing over vegetables.

Top with nuts and feta cheese.

Entrees

Grilled Lamb with Red Raspberry Sauce

(4 servings)

3 pounds lamb or mutton, cut in large chunks

Basil pesto (recipe below)

Wooden grilling skewers

Salt, to taste

Black pepper, to taste

Garlic powder, to taste

Ground rosemary, to taste

Red Raspberry Sauce or **Red Raspberry** Glaze (recipes below)

Flatten pieces of lamb or mutton to approximately ¼ inch thick. Coat with Pesto sauce.

Roll up flattened meat. Place 4 rolls on each wooden grilling skewer. Try to keep sizes uniform.

Cover and refrigerate skewers for at least 2 hours.

Remove from refrigerator and grill over hot charcoals for 20 minutes, until done to liking.

Sprinkle with salt, pepper, **garlic**, and/or ground rosemary to taste (mutton needs more).

Place grilled rolls on a platter and serve with warm **Red Raspberry** Sauce or **Red Raspberry** Glaze (recipes below).

Basil Pesto

¼ cup pine nuts

2 cups fresh **basil** leaves, washed and patted dry

2 cups **Garlic** cloves, peeled and lightly mashed

6 tbsp grated Parmesan cheese

2 tbsp grated Romano cheese

Coarse salt, to taste

½ cup extra-virgin olive oil

Place pine nuts in a dry, heavy skillet and toast over medium-low heat. Remove from skillet and let cool.

Using a food processor, grind **basil** leaves, cooled pine nuts, **Garlic**, both cheeses, and salt to a paste.

Slowly add oil, blending well.

Note: Pesto is best used on the same day, but keeps for three days when its surface is covered with a thin layer of olive oil, and it is tightly covered and chilled.

Red Raspberry Sauce

¼ cup sweet butter

½ cup onion, peeled and chopped onion

¼ cup **carrot**, peeled and chopped

¼ cup chopped celery, minced

2 tbsp flour

1 cup White Zinfandel wine

1 cup strong meat stock or broth

½ cup or more **Red Raspberries**

1 tbsp gourmet mustard

½ tsp lemon juice

1 tsp mixed Italian herbs

Salt, to taste

Fresh ground black pepper, to taste

Heat butter in skillet on medium. Add onion, **carrot**, and celery. Cook until vegetables soften.

Push vegetables to side of pan. Add flour to other side of pan. Mix with butter. Cook for 2 minutes.

Add wine and meat stock. Whisk flour, vegetables, and liquids together to make a smooth sauce. Bring to a simmer and simmer until sauce thickens slightly.

Add **Red Raspberries**, mustard, lemon juice, and herbs. Simmer 2 minutes, stirring gently.

Season with salt and pepper.

Red Raspberry Glaze No. 1

1 cup seedless **Red Raspberry** preserve jam

1 tbsp cornstarch

½ cup White Zinfandel wine

2 tbsp gourmet mustard

Fresh **Red Raspberries**

Lemon zest

Combine jam, cornstarch, wine, and mustard. Stir until cornstarch is dissolved in wine.

Cook in microwave on high approximately 8 minutes or until it thickens.

Add fresh **Red Raspberries** and lemon zest to warm glaze just before serving.

Red Raspberry Chicken

(4 servings)

1 egg
2 tbsp honey
½ cup pecan meal
½ cup whole wheat panko
4 chicken breasts, boneless and skinless
1 tbsp olive oil, as needed
Cooking spray, as needed
Red Raspberry Glaze (recipe below)

In a medium bowl, whisk together egg and honey.

On a plate, mix pecan meal and panko.

Dip chicken in egg mixture, then roll in pecan/panko mixture.

In a large skillet, sauté chicken in olive oil for 10 minutes. Flip chicken and cook 10 more minutes, or until chicken temperature reaches 165 degrees.

To serve, top with **Red Raspberry** glaze.

Red Raspberry Glaze No. 2

½ cup seedless **Red Raspberry** jam
4 tbsp Dijon mustard
2 tbsp balsamic vinegar
1 tsp fresh grated orange peel

In a small saucepan, add jam, mustard, vinegar, and orange peel.

Cook over medium heat for 5 minutes or until glaze consistency is reached. Stir occasionally.

Desserts

Peach Dumplings with Red Raspberry Sauce

(4 servings)

1 refrigerated piecrust

2 peaches, peeled and chopped

Juice from ½ lemon

¼ cup sugar

1 tsp cinnamon

1 tbsp flour

1 egg white, slightly beaten

1 tbsp sugar

½ cup **Red Raspberry** jam

1 tbsp amaretto liqueur

Allow piecrust to stand at room temperature for 15-20 minutes.

Heat oven to 425 degrees.

Cut piecrust into 3-inch squares to yield 8 squares. Reroll dough scraps and cut into squares if needed.

In a small bowl, toss peaches with lemon juice. Add sugar, cinnamon, and flour. Mix gently.

Divide peach mixture among dough squares. Brush dough edges lightly with water. Fold in half, pressing edges to seal.

Brush tops with beaten egg white, then sprinkle with sugar.

Bake for 15-18 minutes.

To make sauce, warm **Red Raspberry** jam in microwave. Add liqueur and mix well.

Serve warm dumplings topped with **Red Raspberry** sauce.

Red Raspberry Cobbler

(4 servings)

½ cup butter, melted
¾ cup milk
1½ cups sugar (divided)
1 cup flour
1½ tsp baking powder
2 cups **Red Raspberries**, fresh or frozen (thawed)

Preheat oven to 350 degrees.
Pour melted butter into bottom of a 7 by 11-inch baking dish.
Mix together milk, 1 cup sugar, flour, and baking powder.
Pour mixture over butter in baking dish. Do not stir.
Pour **Red Raspberries** over batter. Do not stir.
Sprinkle remaining sugar evenly over top of cobbler.
Bake cobbler for 30-45 minutes or until crust is browned.

Red Raspberry Cheesecake

(8 servings)

2 (3-ounce) packages cream cheese, softened
⅔ cup whipping cream
1 (9-inch) baked pastry shell, baked and cooled
1 quart fresh **Red Raspberries**, cleaned (divided)
1 cup sugar
½ cup unsweetened pineapple juice
¼ cup cornstarch
Whipped cream

In a medium bowl, beat together cream cheese and whipping cream.
Spread mix cream cheese mixture over bottom of cooled pie shell. Refrigerate.
Mash half of the **Red Raspberries**. Stir in sugar and let stand for an hour.

Press berry mix through a sieve. Throw away any seeds or solids that remain in sieve.

In a saucepan, mix together pineapple juice, cornstarch, and berry mix. Cook and stir over medium heat until thickened. Let cool.

Reserve ¼ of the thickened berry mix. Spread the rest over cream cheese layer of pie.

Arrange remaining whole **Red Raspberries** over top of pie. Spoon remaining cooked berry mix over whole **Red Raspberries**.

Refrigerate approximately 2 hours or until set.

To serve, top with whipped cream.

Red Raspberry Oatmeal Bars

(18 bars)

1½ cups flour

1 tsp baking powder

¼ tsp salt

½ cup white sugar

½ cup light brown sugar, packed

¾ cup unsalted butter, chilled and cut in pieces

1½ cups quick cooking **Oats**, uncooked

2 cups **Red Raspberries** tossed with 1 cup sugar

½ cup almond slices

Preheat oven to 350 degrees.

Butter a 9-inch square baking pan.

In a large bowl, stir together flour, baking powder, salt, white sugar, and light brown sugar until well blended. Cut in butter until crumbly. Mix in **Oats**.

Press ⅔ of **Oat** mixture into bottom of baking pan.

Spread **Red Raspberries** over oatmeal layer.

Add almonds to remaining **oat** mixture. Sprinkle over **Red Raspberry** layer.

Bake for 30-35 minutes or until golden.

Cool in pan on wire rack, then cut into squares.

Stinging Nettle

Use rubber gloves and tongs — do NOT touch raw plant directly to avoid sting. Cooking the **Stinging Nettles** will remove the stinging properties. If not using fresh **Stinging Nettles**, the freeze-dried version is best. Regularly dried versions may have mold spores that can cause allergic reactions. Fresh leaves and tops are seasonal to spring time. If fresh leaves are not available, you may substitute cut dried, sifted leaves. If the leaves are not sifted, you can sift through a fine metal colander/sieve. Approximately one pound of fresh leaves equals ½ cup of dried sifted leaves. Also, please note that when dried or wilted, **Stinging Nettle** leaves no longer sting.

Stinging Nettle (Urtica dioica and Urtica urens)

Type: Minor galactogogue

Medicinal Dose: 1.8 grams as one (1) 600 mg capsule 3 times a day or 1 cup of tea 2 to 3 times a day; 2 ½ mL to 5 mL of tincture 3 times a day

Other Uses: Mild diuretic and for mild gastrointestinal upset

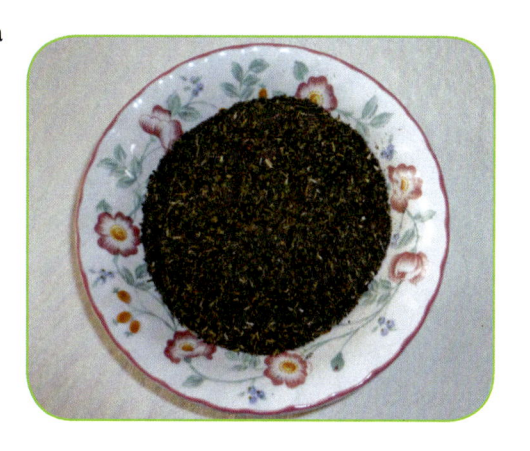

Caution: Stinging nettle may cause mild diuresis and/or mild gastrointestinal upset.

Beverages

Stinging Nettle Tea

(1 serving)

1-2 tsp dried **Stinging Nettles**

8 ounces water

Poor boiling water over **Stinging Nettles** leaves.

Cover and steep for 5-10 minutes.

Strain and serve immediately.

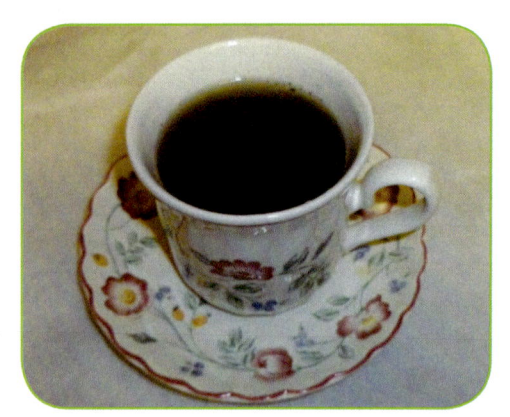

Soups

Dandelion Nettle Soup

(4 servings)

2 tbsp extra-virgin olive oil

1 small onion, chopped

1 small potato, chopped

1 **carrot**, chopped

4 cups **chicken stock**

½ cup dried **Stinging Nettles**

¾ cup (packed) **Dandelion** greens (parboil 5-10 minutes to remove bitterness)

¼ cup watercress, chopped

¼ cup **spinach**, chopped

2 tbsp butter

Croutons, as desired

Heat oil in a pan. Sauté onion, potato, and **carrots** until onion is translucent.

Add stock and bring to a boil. Simmer until potato and **carrots** are tender.

Add **Stinging Nettle**, **Dandelion**, watercress, and **spinach**. Simmer for 15 minutes.

Add butter.

Using an immersion blender, blend until soup is smooth.

To serve, top with croutons.

Irish Stinging Nettle Soup

(1 serving)

2 tbsp butter

¼ cup **Oatmeal**

10 fluid ounces water, **chicken stock**, or low-fat milk

2 young, tender **Stinging Nettle** tops, washed and minced (use rubber gloves and tongs)

Salt, to taste

Ground black pepper, to taste

Heat butter in pot. Sprinkle in **Oatmeal** and fry until golden. Stir in water, stock, or milk. Bring to a boil, stirring constantly.

Add **Stinging Nettles**, salt, and pepper.

Bring to a boil. Lower heat and simmer for 30-45 minutes.

Stinging Nettle Soup 1

(4 servings)

1 pound fresh **Stinging Nettles**, washed and chopped (wear rubber gloves and use tongs)

2 tbsp extra-virgin olive oil

1 white onion, diced

4 cups **chicken broth**

1 pound **rice**, cooked

Salt, to taste

Ground black pepper, to taste

Bring a large pot of salted water to a boil. Add **Stinging Nettles** and cook for 1-2 minutes, until softened. Drain in colander and rinse with cold water.

Heat olive oil in a large pot over medium-low heat. Stir in onion and cook until onion is translucent.

Add **chicken broth** and **Stinging Nettles**. Bring to a boil. Reduce heat, cover, and simmer for 15 minutes.

Using an immersion blender, puree soup.

Serve over cooked **rice** seasoned with salt and pepper.

Stinging Nettle Soup 2

(1 serving)

10 ounces beef broth

2 young tender **Stinging Nettles** tops, rinsed and finely chopped (wear rubber gloves and use tongs)

3 tbsp flour

2 tbsp margarine or butter, melted

Salt, to taste

Ground white pepper, to taste

1 tsp parsley

Chives, finely minced

2 hardboiled eggs, cut in half, or poached eggs

Bring beef broth to a boil. Add **Stinging Nettles** and cook until tender.

In a small bowl, stir together flour and margarine or butter. Add to soup and cook until soup thickens.

Add salt, pepper, parsley, and chives.

Serve with hardboiled or poached eggs.

Entrees

Gnocchi Verde (Green Dumplings)

(4-6 servings)

10 ounces frozen **spinach**, thawed and liquid removed

1½ tsp salt (divided)

2 ounces bacon

2 **Garlic** cloves, chopped, to taste (divided)

1 small onion, chopped

1 egg

1 cup ricotta cheese

½ cup flour, plus additional flour for thickening and dusting

½ cup **Stinging Nettles** leaves, cut, dried, and sifted

½ cup grated Parmesan cheese (divided)

1 tbsp butter

2 tbsp rum (or substitute)

2 large tomatoes, chopped

1 cup baked beans

¼ tsp nutmeg

½ tsp ground black pepper

½ tsp oregano

Preheat oven to 350 degrees.

Steam **spinach** with 1 tsp salt for 5 minutes until compacted. Remove from heat, drain, and squeeze **spinach** to remove any excess liquid.

In a large skillet, fry bacon. Add 1 clove **Garlic** and onion. Cook until onion is translucent. Stir to keep **Garlic** from burning.

In a large bowl, whisk together egg and salt. Beat in ricotta cheese and flour. Add **spinach**, bacon mixture, **Stinging Nettles**, and ¼ cup Parmesan cheese. Mix well. If needed, add additional flour to form dough.

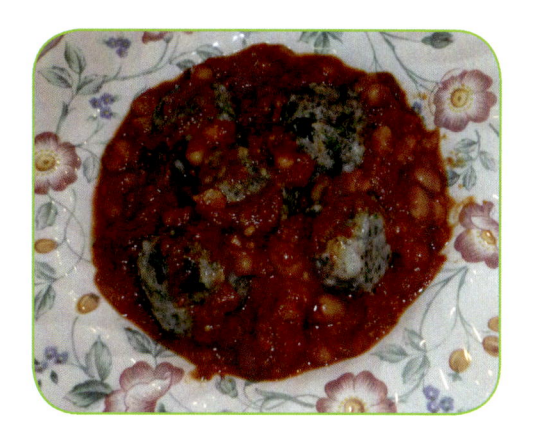

Flour a large surface. Roll out dough approximately 1 inch thick. Cut into 1-inch squares. Roll into balls, dust with flour, and place in a buttered ovenproof pan.

Bake for 20 minutes.

Sauté 1 clove **Garlic** in melted butter in a large pot. Add rum, tomatoes, and baked beans. Cook until thickened.

In a small bowl, mix together ¼ cup Parmesan cheese, nutmeg, black pepper, and oregano.

To serve, top dumplings with bean sauce and garnish with Parmesan cheese mixture.

Ravioli with Stinging Nettle Sauce

(4-6 servings)

⅔ cup ricotta cheese

½ cup grated Parmesan cheese + additional for garnish

32 pieces wonton skin squares

Rice flour to dust tray

Stinging Nettle sauce (recipe below)

½ cup pine nuts, roasted

In a bowl, mix ricotta and Parmesan cheese together.

Lay out wonton skin squares.

On each square, place 1 tsp of Ricotta cheese mixture in center of each square. Brush edges lightly with water. Bring opposite corners to meet, forming a triangle. Press edges lightly to seal. Place on a baking tray dusted with **rice** flour.

Bring a large pot of salted water to boil. Gently drop in half the raviolis. Cook until they float to top. Remove and drain. Repeat with rest of ravioli.

Spoon **Stinging Nettle** sauce over cooked ravioli.

Sprinkle with pine nuts and grated Parmesan cheese.

Stinging Nettle Sauce

1 pound fresh **Stinging Nettles**, chopped or ½ cup dried

2 tbsp butter

2 **Garlic** cloves, thinly sliced

½ cup heavy cream

1 tsp salt

½ tsp black pepper, cracked

In a skillet, melt butter over medium high heat. Sauté **Garlic** until tender.

Add fresh **Stinging Nettles**. Cover and cook until wilted. If using dried **Stinging Nettle**, stir in with **Garlic**.

Add cream, salt, and pepper. Cook on medium heat until liquid reduces to half.

Using an immersion blender, puree until smooth. Keep warm until ravioli is ready.

Stinging Nettle Mashed Potatoes

(2 servings)

1½ pounds potatoes, chopped

1 small onion, chopped

2 young tender **Stinging Nettle** tops, washed and finely chopped (wear rubber gloves and use tongs)

1 cup milk

Salt, to taste

Freshly ground black pepper, to taste

4 tbsp butter

Boil potatoes and onion until soft. Drain. Return to saucepan and mash.

While potatoes and onions are cooking, bring **Stinging Nettle** and milk to a boil in another saucepan. Gently boil for 10 minutes. Milk will curdle (this is OK).

Fold **Stinging Nettle** mixture into mashed potatoes. Season with salt and pepper.

Warm on low heat for a few minutes, stirring to dry mixture a little.

To serve, put mixture in serving bowl. Top with butter.

Stinging Nettle Pasta

(4 servings)

  8 ounces spicy Italian sausage

  1 tbsp **Fennel** seeds, cut into ¼-inch pieces

  1 pound **Stinging Nettles**, rinsed (use rubber gloves and tongs) and chopped (or ½ cup dried)

  4 cups (approximately 1/2 pound) kale, finely minced

  ½ cup **chicken stock**

  4 servings green pasta, cooked

  2 tsp salt plus salt, to taste

  Freshly ground black pepper, to taste

  ½ cup grated Parmesan cheese

In a large skillet, cook sausage and **Fennel** seeds over low heat until fat begins to melt. Turn heat up to medium and cook until most fat from sausage has cooked out and sausage is golden brown.

Add **Stinging Nettles**, kale, and **chicken stock**. Cook until greens are very soft. Season with salt and pepper.

Add cooked pasta, stirring to coat. Cook a few minutes to warm pasta.

Add grated Parmesan cheese. Toss to mix.

Serve.

Sides

Stinging Nettle Custard

(4 servings)

  1 leek (thinly chop tender white end only)

  2 **Garlic** cloves, thinly sliced

  2 tbsp olive oil

  4 cups **Stinging Nettle** leaves, washed and

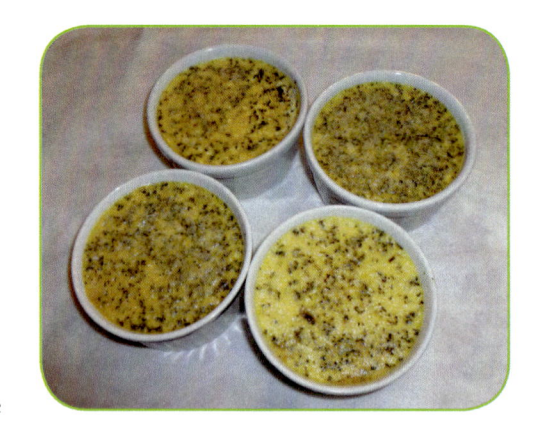

chopped (use rubber gloves and tongs)

3 eggs plus 2 egg yolks, at room temperature

½ teaspoon salt

1 cup grated Parmesan cheese

¾ cup milk

1¾ cups cream

Preheat oven to 300 degrees.

Sauté leeks and **Garlic** in olive oil under tender.

Add **Stinging Nettle**. Sauté until tender. Cool, then put in a cloth and wring out all liquid.

Butter four 4-inch soufflé dishes. Put ¼ **Stinging Nettle** mixture into bottom of each soufflé dish.

Place soufflé dishes in a large baking dish (deep enough to hold custards' water bath) and space soufflé dishes at least 1 inch apart.

Gently warm milk and cream in a small saucepan. Let cool.

In a large bowl, whisk eggs, yolks, and salt until blended. Add grated Parmesan cheese. Slowly pour milk mixture into egg mixture, whisking continuously.

Pour ¼ egg cream mixture into each soufflé dish to cover **Stinging Nettle** mixture.

Pour hot (NOT boiling) water into large baking dish holding custard soufflé dishes. Water should reach 1 inch below rims of soufflé dishes.

Put in oven and bake for approximately 35 minutes. To test for doneness, carefully tilt a soufflé dish to side. If center bulges, but no liquid leaks out, custard is done.

Serve warm or at room temperature.

Stinging Nettle with Nuts

(2 servings)

2 onions, finely chopped

4 tbsp vegetable oil

½ cup **rice**

Cayenne pepper, to taste

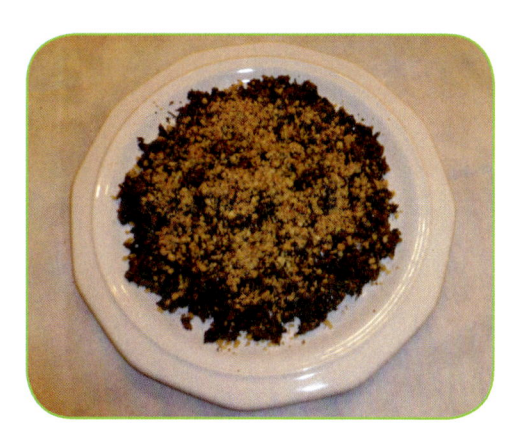

1 pound fresh **Stinging Nettle**, washed and chopped (wear rubber gloves and use tongs)

Salt, to taste

⅓ cup walnuts, ground

In a large skillet, sauté onions in oil until translucent. Add **rice** and cayenne pepper. Sauté until **rice** is slightly browned.

Add **Stinging Nettles**.

Add just enough hot water to cover **Stinging Nettles**. Bring to a boil, then simmer for 30 minutes. Mixture should be thick.

Season with salt to taste.

To serve, dish into bowls and top with walnuts.

Thistles

There is some confusion as to whether **Milk Thistle** and **Blessed Thistle** are the same or different forms of the herbal. They are entirely two different plants. Other "**Thistles**" may also be effective galactogogues.

Blessed Thistle (Cnici benedicti herba)

Type: Major galactogogue

Medicinal Dose: Up to 2 grams, in capsule form, daily

Other Uses: May increase appetite and settle upset stomach

Caution: Blessed Thistle may cause allergic reaction.

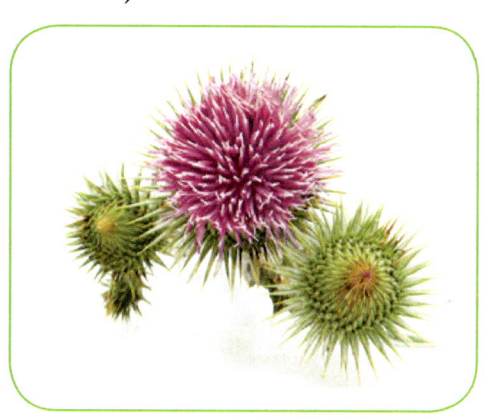

Milk Thistle (Cardui mariae herba)

Type: Major galactogogue

Medicinal Dose: 12 grams to 15 grams daily as infusion (equal to 200 mg to 400 mg of silibinin)

Use: For possible liver protective properties

Caution: Milk thistle may have laxative effect and/or cause allergic reaction.

Beverages

Blessed Thistle Tea

(1 serving; herbal remedy)

1 cup water

1-2 tsp dried loose **Blessed Thistle** or 1 dried **Blessed Thistle** teabag

Bring water to a boil, then remove from heat.

Add **Blessed Thistle** teabag or dried loose **Blessed Thistle**, and let steep for 5 minutes.

Remove teabag or strain loose herbs before drinking.

Milk Thistle and Red Raspberry Smoothie

(1 serving)

1 tsp **Milk Thistle** seeds, finely ground (or liquid extract)

1 cup **Red Raspberries**, frozen

1 cup milk, cold

1 cup **Red Raspberry** yogurt

2 tbsp honey

1 ripe banana, peeled and frozen

¼ tsp vanilla

6-8 ice cubes

Cover ground **Milk Thistle** seeds with warm water and soak overnight.

Place **Red Raspberries** and ½ cup milk in blender. Blend on high until smooth.

Add remaining milk, **Red Raspberry** yogurt, honey, banana, vanilla, and **Milk Thistle** seeds (including water) or liquid extract. Blend until smooth.

Add crushed ice cubes and blend until smooth.

Milk Thistle Seed Tea

(1 serving)

2 tsp **Milk Thistle** seeds

1 ounce chamomile flowers

1 cup boiling water

Crush **Milk Thistle** seeds with a mortar and pestle or in coffee grinder.

In teapot, put ground **Milk Thistle** seeds and chamomile flowers. Add boiling water.

Let sit for 30 minutes.

Strain into cup.

Breakfasts

Milk Thistle Muesli

(12 servings)

1 cup **flax seeds**, ground

1 cup **Milk Thistle** seeds, ground

4 cups rolled **Oats**

2 cups **Oat** bran

½ cup dried fruit (raisins, dates, cranberries, blueberries…)

1 cup **sunflower seeds** and/or **pumpkin** seeds (can be ground)

1 cup almonds

1 cup lecithin granules

½ cup chia seeds (optional)

1 tsp spices (**Coriander**, **Fennel**, **turmeric**, **Ginger**, cinnamon, and/or other herbs/spices)

Water, milk, almond milk, soy milk, **rice** milk, or apple juice

Red Raspberries

Mix dry ingredients together. Store in refrigerator.

To prepare to serve, place 1 cup dry mix in a bowl with a lid. Add enough milk or juice to cover dry mix. Cover bowl and let sit in refrigerator overnight.

When ready to serve, add additional milk or juice, if needed, and top with **Red Raspberries**.

Milk Thistle Porridge

(1 serving)

½ cup **Milk Thistle** seeds

¼ cup **flax seeds**

3-4 dried apricots and/or mangos, sliced

1 tbsp agave nectar or sugar

1 tsp cinnamon powder

Cover **Milk Thistle** seeds with warm water, and soak overnight. Drain.

Cover **flax seeds** with ½ cup warm water, and soak overnight. Drain.

Cover apricots or mangos with warm water, and soak overnight. Drain, reserving liquid.

Place seeds and apricots or mangos in a food processor with an "S" blade. Process until a thick porridge is achieved, adding reserved liquid from apricots or mangos if needed.

Put in cereal bowl. Add agave or sugar and cinnamon, and mix well.

Condiments

Milk Thistle Condiment

(Several spice jars)

½ ounce wild nori (or **seaweed** of choice)

1½ cups **sesame seeds**

¼ cup **Milk Thistle** seeds

¼ cup salt

Preheat oven to 300 degrees. Arrange nori flat on a cookie sheet. Bake until toasty, approximately 10-15 minutes. Break into small pieces and grind in a spice or coffee grinder until very small.

Dry-roast **sesame seeds** in a skillet over medium-high heat, turning frequently. Seeds are ready when fragrant and slightly darkened. Allow to cool.

Grind **Milk Thistle** seeds in coffee or spice grinder until very small.

In a medium bowl, combine **seaweed**, **sesame seeds**, **Milk Thistle**, and salt. Mix well.

Place mixture in clean spice jars. Put lids on jars and store in a cool, dark cabinet or pantry. Use within a month or two, as the oil in the seeds will become rancid with extended storage.

Vervain

Note that **Vervain** is contraindicated in pregnancy due to its oxytocic properties. It is not contraindicated in breastfeeding.

Vervain (Verbena officinalis)

Type: Minor galactogogue

Medicinal Dose: 30 grams to 50 grams daily as tea

Use: For anxiety and hypertension

Caution: Do not use if pregnant due to oxytocic (uterine stimulant) properties.

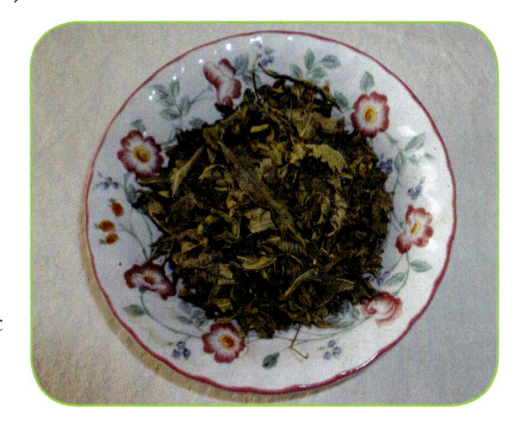

Beverages

Vervain Mint Tea

(4 servings; herbal remedy)

1 quart water
½ cup fresh mint leaves, rinsed and lightly packed
½ cup fresh **Vervain** leaves, rinsed and lightly packed

Bring water to a boil.

Place mint and **Vervain** leaves in a teapot. Pour hot water over leaves.

Let steep approximately 3-5 minutes. Strain and serve.

Vervain Tea

(4 servings)

1 cup fresh **Vervain** leaves
1 quart water

Bring water to a boil, turn off heat. Add **Vervain** leaves, cover, and let steep 5 minutes.

Uncover and allow to cool for a few minutes.

Strain and serve.

Desserts

Peach Vervain Tart

(6-8 servings)

Vervain-Infused Custard Base
1½ cups milk
20 **Vervain** fresh leaves or 4 **Vervain** tea bags
2 egg yolks

2 tbsp cornstarch

¼ cup sugar

¼ cup ground almonds

In a saucepan, bring milk to a boil milk.

Add **Vervain** leaves or contents of tea bags.

Turn off heat, cover saucepan, and let **Vervain** steep for 15 minutes.

In a medium bowl, mix together egg yolks, cornstarch, sugar, and ground almonds.

Strain **Vervain**-infused milk. Blend into egg mixture slowly.

Return mixture to saucepan and reheat to just boiling. Lower heat and cook until mixture becomes thick. Stirring frequently.

Set aside to cool.

Cream Topping

1 cup whipping cream

¼ cup sugar

¼ cup ground almonds

1 plum, 1 peach, 1 nectarine, and/or any ripened fruit, chopped

Whip cream until stiff, adding sugar halfway.

Fold in ground almonds.

Fold in chopped fruit.

Refrigerate.

Tart

Pastry crust in prepared pie pan

Vervain-infused custard (recipe above)

2 large peaches, sliced in half moon shape

2 tsp sugar

Cream topping (recipe above)

Fresh **Vervain** leaves, as garnish

Pierce pastry crust with a fork and place in freezer for 30 minutes (this will prevent dough from shrinking when baked).

Preheat oven to 350 degrees.

Line inside of pastry crust with parchment paper. Bake for 15 minutes.

Remove crust from oven and remove parchment paper.

Fill base of crust with custard. Top with sliced peaches, placed next to each other, with one end on the edge of the crust and the other facing the center. Press peaches in slightly and sprinkle with sugar

Return to oven and bake for 20 minutes.

Remove from oven and let cool completely. (The peaches might get watery, but will set nicely once cooled down.)

To serve, top with cream topping and garnish with fresh **Vervain** leaves.

References

Blumenthal, M., Busse, W. R., Goldberg, A., & Gruenwald, J., et al, Eds. (1998). *The complete German commission e monographs: therapeutic guide to herbal medicines.* Austin, TX: American Botanical Council.

Hale, T. W. (2012). *Medications and mother's milk, 15th ed.* Amarillo: Hale Publishing.

Humphrey, S. (2007). Herbal therapies during lactation. In: Hale, T., Hartmann, P., eds. *Textbook of human lactation.* Amarillo TX: Hale Publishing.

Humphrey, S. (2003). *Nursing mother's herbal.* Minneapolis MN: Fairview Press.

Marasco, L. (2008). ILCA's inside track: A resource for breastfeeding mothers: Increasing your milk supply with galactogogues. *J Hum Lact*, 24(4):455-6.

Nice, F. J. (2011). *Nonprescription drugs for the breastfeeding mother, 2nd ed.* Amarillo: Hale Publishing; 2011.

Nice, F. J., Coghlan, R. J., & Birmingham, B. T. (2000). Herbals and breastfeeding. *US Pharmacist*, 25:28, 31-2, 34, 41-2, 45-6.

PDR for nonprescription drugs, dietary supplements, and herbs, 32nd ed. (2011). Montvale: PDR Network, LLC.

To access techniques, tools, and information on the use of herbals and galactogogues and to download articles, please visit my website: www.nicebreastfeeding.com

Index

A

Alfalfa 35, 36, 37, 39, 40, 41, 42, 44, 45
Almonds 147, 162, 191, 192, 193, 199, 219, 226, 232, 245
Anise 47, 48, 49, 50, 51, 52, 53, 54, 55, 56, 57, 58, 59, 146, 153, 209
Asparagus 44, 112, 113

B

Barley 61
Basil 41, 56, 72, 112, 131, 139, 142, 145, 146, 170, 227
Beer 62, 63, 64, 65, 66, 67, 69, 70, 71, 72, 82
Beets 40, 140, 226
Borage 96, 113, 117, 147

C

Caraway 75, 76, 77, 79, 80, 82, 83, 84, 85, 87, 88, 89, 152
Carrots 37, 40, 49, 53, 66, 71, 78, 82, 89, 98, 99, 112, 128, 143, 167, 170, 172, 179, 191, 226, 228, 234
Chasteberry 91, 92
Cherries 175, 191, 199
Chicken Broth 41, 53, 73, 98, 134, 143, 147, 160
Chicken Stock 49, 66, 99, 102, 105, 112, 167, 170, 240
Chickpeas 36, 45, 83, 166, 226
Coconut 97, 155, 184, 186, 187, 192
Coriander 45, 68, 87, 88, 95, 97, 99, 100, 101, 102, 103, 104, 106, 110, 146, 152, 153, 155, 159, 160, 167, 245

Cumin 97, 100, 101, 102, 106, 140, 152, 153, 155, 156, 157, 159, 161, 167, 171, 176, 194

D

Dandelion 109, 110, 112, 113, 114, 115, 116, 117, 118, 119, 120, 234
Dill 40, 44, 121, 122, 123, 124, 125, 126, 127, 128, 129, 130, 131, 132, 133, 134, 145, 168, 178, 196, 221

F

Fennel 54, 59, 106, 135, 136, 137, 138, 139, 140, 142, 143, 144, 145, 146, 147, 148, 149, 153, 155, 156, 161, 240, 245
Fenugreek 151, 152, 153, 154, 155, 156, 157, 159, 160, 161, 162
Flax Seeds 245, 246

G

Garlic 41, 50, 51, 54, 55, 63, 64, 65, 66, 67, 70, 71, 72, 80, 83, 86, 87, 99, 101, 103, 105, 106, 111, 112, 113, 114, 116, 117, 124, 129, 130, 131, 137, 138, 139, 140, 145, 146, 147, 148, 152, 155, 156, 157, 158, 160, 166, 167, 168, 169, 170, 171, 172, 173, 174, 175, 176, 177, 178, 179, 194, 195, 197, 220, 225, 227, 237, 238, 240
Ginger 43, 50, 51, 52, 53, 55, 70, 83, 87, 97, 100, 105, 106, 147, 152, 155, 156, 157, 160, 196, 220, 245
Goat's Rue 181, 182
Green Beans 39, 112, 114, 170

H

Hibiscus 184
Hops 61

L

Lemon Balm 216
Lentils 98, 220
Lettuce 38, 39, 40, 41, 42, 48, 103, 127, 129, 226

M

Marshmallow Root 183, 184, 186, 187
Molasses (Black Strap) 66, 171
Mung 220
Mushrooms 37, 45, 52, 53, 130, 143, 147

O

Oat 77, 190, 191, 192, 193, 194, 196, 197, 198, 200, 201, 202, 235, 245

P

Peas 83, 112, 126, 172, 179, 204, 221
Pumpkin 133
Pumpkin Seeds 245

Q

Quinoa 178

R

Red Clover 215, 216, 217, 218, 219, 220, 221
Red Raspberries 92, 194, 219, 223, 224, 225, 226, 228, 229, 230, 231, 232, 244
Rice 54, 73, 80, 83, 87, 136, 187, 235, 241
Rice 238

S

Seaweed 204, 246
Sesame Seeds 42, 166, 246
Spinach 39, 40, 49, 98, 113, 115, 136, 155, 219, 226, 234, 237
Stinging Nettles 233, 234, 235, 236, 238, 240, 242
Sunflower Seeds 37, 245
Sweet Potato 99

T

Thistle 243, 244, 245, 246
Turmeric 49, 87, 97, 99, 105, 115, 152, 153, 154, 155, 157, 160, 161, 245

V

Vervain 249, 250

About the Authors

Frank J. Nice, Pharmacist

Frank J. Nice has practiced as a Polish cook, consultant, lecturer, and author on medications and breastfeeding for over 40 years. He holds a Bachelor's Degree in Pharmacy, a Masters Degree in Pharmacy Administration, and Masters and Doctorate Degrees in Public Administration. Dr. Nice holds Certification in Public Health Pharmacy and is registered as a pharmacist in Pennsylvania, Maine, Arizona, and Maryland.

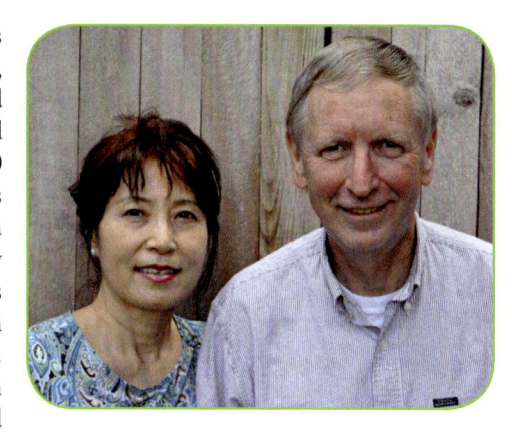

Dr. Nice has organized and participated in over three dozen medical missions to the country of Haiti. He retired from the US Public Health Service after 30 years of distinguished service as a Commissioned Officer and pharmacist. He continues to work full time as a pharmacist and grandfather to many grandchildren all over the country.

Myung Hee Nice

Myung Hee Nice has practiced as a Korean cook for over 40 years. She holds a Bachelor's Degree in English Literature and a Masters Degree in Information Technology.

Myung provides at home support for Frank while he is in Haiti and feeds him while he is at home. She continues to work part time in the information technology field and full time as a grandmother to numerous grandchildren, present and to come.

Ordering Information

Hale Publishing, L.P.
1825 E. Plano Parkway
Suite 280
Plano, TX 75074

8:00 a.m. to 5:00 p.m. CST

Call » 972.578.0400
Fax » 972.578.0413

Online
www.ibreastfeeding.com